RAND
CORPORATION

The Public Health Impacts of Gaza's Water Crisis

Analysis and Policy Options

Shira Efron, Jordan R. Fischbach, Ilana Blum, Rouslan I. Karimov, Melinda Moore

For more information on this publication, visit www.rand.org/t/RR2515

Library of Congress Cataloging-in-Publication Data is available for this publication.
ISBN: 978-1-9774-0163-2

Published by the RAND Corporation, Santa Monica, Calif.

Cover: REUTERS/Ibraheem Abu Mustafa

Preface

Gaza has long suffered from a dual water crisis: a shortage of potable water for drinking, cooking, and hygiene, combined with a lack of wastewater sanitation. In addition, more than 108,000 cubic meters of untreated sewage flow daily from Gaza into the Mediterranean Sea, creating extreme public health hazards in Gaza, Israel, and Egypt. While these problems are not new, rapidly deteriorating infrastructure, strict limitations on the importation of construction materials and water pumps, and a diminished and unreliable energy supply have in recent years accelerated the water crisis and exacerbated the water-related health risks.

This report describes the relationship between Gaza's water problems and its energy challenges and examines the implications of Gaza's water crisis for public health. It reviews the state of the current domestic water supply and state of water sanitation in Gaza and analyzes water-related risks to public health in Gaza and potential risks for Israel and Egypt. The report then recommends a number of steps to ameliorate the crisis and decrease the potential for a regional public health disaster that take into consideration current political constraints. The audience for this report includes stakeholders involved in Gaza, including the Palestinian, Israeli, and Egyptian governments, various international organizations and nongovernmental organizations working on the ground there, and the donor community seeking to rehabilitate the region. The report should also be valuable to academics and experts assessing the current status of Gaza's humanitarian crisis and its possible effects if unaddressed.

This report was funded through the generous contributions of the RAND Center for Middle East Public Policy (CMEPP) Advisory Board and conducted within CMEPP, part of International Programs at the RAND Corporation.

RAND Ventures

RAND is a research organization that develops solutions to public policy challenges to help make communities throughout the world safer and more secure, healthier and more prosperous. RAND is nonprofit, nonpartisan, and committed to the public interest. RAND Ventures is a vehicle for investing in policy solutions. Philanthropic contributions support our ability to take the long view, tackle tough and often-controversial topics, and share our findings in innovative and compelling ways. RAND's research findings and recommendations are based on data and evidence, and therefore do not necessarily reflect the policy preferences or interests of its clients, donors, or supporters. Funding for this venture was provided by gifts from RAND supporters and income from operations.

RAND Center for Middle East Public Policy

This work was conducted within the RAND Center for Middle East Public Policy (CMEPP). CMEPP brings together analytic excellence and regional expertise from across the RAND Corporation to address the most critical political, social, and economic challenges facing the Middle East today. For more information about the RAND Center for Middle East Public Policy, visit www.rand.org/cmepp or contact the director (contact information is provided on the webpage).

Contents

Figures and Table

Figures

Table

Summary

Gaza has long had water and sanitation challenges, but today it is in a state of emergency. The main source of water—its aquifer—is being depleted and its quality diminished by seawater intrusion, wastewater seepage, and agricultural runoff. Gaza's inconsistent energy supply hinders the operation of Gaza's existing water facilities and prevents the construction of new ones. With insufficient potable water, Gaza residents lack water not only for drinking but also for hygiene and sanitation. More than a quarter of all reported disease in Gaza is caused by poor water quality and access. If present trends continue, Gaza and the surrounding region are at risk of a disease outbreak or other public health crises.

While these problems are not new for Gaza, RAND's analysis shows that a recent confluence of events has exacerbated the situation to a point of great urgency. Recurring conflict with Israel has severely damaged Gaza's infrastructure for water, sanitation, and hygiene, but Israel's and Egypt's restrictions on border access and the movement of goods have hampered repairs. Israel has for years restricted the imports of "dual-use" items that could be used for both civilian and military purposes—including 70 percent of the technical equipment (e.g., pumps, water purification chemicals) that is needed to maintain water and sanitation. Furthermore, Gaza's power supply, always in deficit, has since 2017 been subjected to an intra-Palestinian dispute over electricity payments between the Palestinian Authority (PA) and Hamas, Gaza's de facto government. This dispute, combined with wrecked infrastructure, has left Gaza's residents with only some four hours of electricity per day, far from sufficient to support basic living standards.

In addition, international funding to support urgent humanitarian interventions, finalize reconstruction, and revitalize the private sector economy has been limited. This includes medium- to long-term infrastructure projects in the energy; water, sanitation, and hygiene (WASH); and public health sectors. For example, as of late March 2018, a funding gap of $244 million was cited as hindering reconstruction from the 2014 war, including damage to homes, hospitals, and water and energy infrastructure. International donors made $3.5 billion pledges for reconstruction after the war, but half of these funds have not been disbursed. This example highlights one of the most challenging funding aspects related to Gaza—a lack of donor follow-through. Moreover, the 2017 $547 million Humanitarian Response Plan for the Palestinian Territories, most of it geared toward Gaza, was less than 50 percent funded, with the WASH portion particularly underfunded.

The United States recently decided to cut $300 million in funding this year intended for the UN Relief and Works Agency (UNRWA) for Palestine Refugees in the Near East on grounds that the organization needs to reform and that other donors should step in. This decision could further worsen the situation, especially as Gaza's hospitals are becoming increasingly inoperable. UNRWA supports the WASH sector and provides public health services in Gaza, operating 21 primary health clinics, employing more than 1,000 medical staff, serving more than 4 million annual patient visits, and running schools where some WASH educational programs are taught. In addition to slashing UNRWA funding, the U.S. government also cut $200 million in bilateral foreign aid that was designated for humanitarian programs in the West Bank and Gaza.

Major future projects are also hindered by funding gaps. For example, the Gaza Central Desalination Plant, which is expected to provide 139 million cubic meters (mcm) of water per year by 2023, still needed some $120 million to $230 million to begin construction as of March 2018. Completed infrastructure projects also suffer from underfunding. For instance, the Northern Gaza Emergency Sewage

Treatment (NGEST) became operational in early 2018, but there is a $16.8 million funding gap for NGEST to cover operation and maintenance costs (donors are willing to fund infrastructure projects but not operation and maintenance), hindering its ability to provide wastewater treatment for more than 400,000 of North Gaza's residents.

To be sure, the funding shortage and lack of funders' follow-through are not the only challenges preventing the rehabilitation of Gaza's energy, water, and health sectors. More than anything, the water-energy-health crisis in Gaza represents a failure of governance. Indeed, the key underlying problems could be fully addressed in the long term through greater investment in water and wastewater treatment infrastructure and new power infrastructure, along with greater water or electricity purchases from outside Gaza. These are all achievable with existing technologies but are hindered for political reasons. Thus, all stakeholders should strive to find politically feasible solutions, including working with the PA and regional and international mediators. At the same time, it is necessary to relax restrictions on access and movement of goods necessary for the water, energy, and health sectors and to address other implementation challenges, as detailed next.

What Can Be Done to Lower the Risk of a Waterborne Health Crisis in Gaza?

Given the significant challenges at the intersection of water, energy, and public health in Gaza, RAND researchers analyzed how improving each of these critical sectors would help ameliorate the waterborne risks to Gaza residents. This analysis draws on a variety of sources, including reports by governments and international organizations, policy papers by think tanks and research institutes, media and news reports, and off-the-record conversations with current and former Israeli and Palestinian government officials and diverse experts from the United Nations, World Health Organization (WHO), the Office of the Quartet (an organization that includes the United Nations, United States, European Union, and Russia), and nongovernmental organizations.

We identified a number of near- and long-term steps—some of which are already under way but at risk of being undermined due to political tensions—that would address many challenges in the areas of power and water infrastructure and public health. We recognize, however, that implementation issues that stem from the region's complex political context defy easy solutions. Based on our analysis, we make the following recommendations.

Increase the Quantity and Consistency of Gaza's Electricity Supply

Without a consistent supply of fuel and electricity, Gaza's capacity to operate its existing desalination, freshwater, and wastewater treatment plants and build new ones is severely limited. The following recommendations are aimed at increasing the quantity and consistency of power:

- Advance the "161kV Line"—a high-voltage connection between Gaza and the Israel Electric Corporation grid—that would add 100 megawatts (MW) per day within a few years. Israel and the PA have in principle agreed to establishing this connection, yet the agreement has not been finalized, and funding is lacking.
- Increase power supply from Egypt. An additional 25 MW per day could be available by mid-2019, according to the Quartet.
- Upgrade and expand the electricity transmission network to Gaza and its internal distribution network to enable additional and diverse domestic generation capacity and imports. A first step should be rehabilitating the connection with Egypt, which has been unreliable.
- Restore the fuel storage tank at the Gaza Power Plant (GPP) to enable more sustainable operation.
- Connect the GPP to a natural gas supply pipeline, which would allow it to operate at its maximum capacity of 140 MW per day (increased from the 0 to 25 MW produced as of mid-2018 at a substantially lower cost). In the longer term, connect Gaza more broadly to Israel's natural gas infrastructure to support new gas-fired power plants. Gas-based power generation for Gaza could increase to some 600 MW per day.

- Ensure a reliable power supply to the NGEST plant.
- Supply the 1.5 MW required to operate the Khan Yunis Short-Term Low-Volume (STLV) desalination plant for 22 hours per day, which would provide potable water to the 75,000 residents of Khan Yunis and Rafah.
- Invest in new solar energy projects, which could make lifeline infrastructure more resilient.
- Improve fee collection and mediate intra-Palestinian arrangements to ensure that these fees are used to cover the ongoing cost of Gaza electricity.
- Advance development of the Gaza Marine gas field, located 20 miles off the Gaza coast and estimated to hold more than 1 trillion cubic feet of natural gas.

Increase the Potable Water Supply and Improve Wastewater Treatment

Several of the recommendations that follow depend on resolving Gaza's inconsistent supply of fuel and electricity but also concern other issues:

- Augment the potable water supply by increasing water purchases from Israel. Israel and the PA should advance the finalization, and then the implementation, of the previously agreed-upon Red Sea–Dead Sea project between Israel and the PA, which is designed to provide additional quantities of potable water to Gaza (and the West Bank).
- Increase desalination capacity, allowing for additional treatment of raw water at the industrial or household scale.
- Advance plans to begin construction of the Gaza Central Desalination Plant, which will initially provide 55 mcm of potable water yearly. To do so, donors should help close the remaining $230 million funding gap, and Israel and the PA, with the support of the international community, should agree on the terms for entry of construction materials into Gaza.
- Improve the water storage and distribution system in Gaza. Additional storage would allow Gaza to purchase more water, and

repairing the transmission and distribution pipes would prevent water loss to leakage and ensure that treated water reaches residents.
- Invest in various wastewater treatment methods to eliminate exposure to raw sewage and the incidence of waterborne hazards.
- Distribute chemicals and spare parts for existing household treatment systems, including materials on Israel's dual-use list, to prevent outbreaks of waterborne disease.
- Construct more wastewater treatment plants, including the three or more projects that are already under way. Ensure that the funding gap for NGEST is closed and that the PA finalizes plans for sustained operations.
- Consider using treated wastewater to recharge the coastal aquifer (indirect potable reuse) or as a primary source for potable water (direct potable reuse). The former could also potentially prevent further seawater intrusion and reduce chloride and nitrogen levels.
- Repair the wastewater collection system to reduce the flow of untreated sewage into surface waters and groundwater and connect the remaining third of Gaza residents who lack access and now use cesspits and open drains.

Protect Public Health and Promote Hygiene and Sanitation Practices

International funding plays a significant role in protecting public health in Gaza and preventing the spread of disease. The following list includes recommendations for Gaza's global support system:

- Prevent and prepare for disease outbreaks, including by providing cholera vaccinations and World Health Organization/United Nations Children's Fund rehydration salt packets to Gaza residents.
- Maintain basic health services in Gaza, including through international funding for clinics and physicians (e.g., UNRWA), sustaining the energy supply to hospitals (including by guaranteeing emergency fuel supplies are available), and ensuring that sanitation and hygiene are maintained in medical facilities.

- Promote more-rigorous hygiene and sanitation education in general, and especially in schools. Students, as the most vulnerable age group for waterborne diseases, also require better access to safe drinking water and sanitation facilities.
- Create a regional pandemic task force to prevent a disease outbreak and implement containment.

Reduce Import Barriers and Work Within Political Differences

The current barriers to policy solutions are largely political. While there is a need to address these political issues and reach practical arrangements that will enable the PA to assume responsibility for managing Gaza's affairs, we also recommend that regional and international stakeholders render the following assistance:

- Capitalize on the commitments of donors who pledged funds for major WASH projects through the creation of a follow-up mechanism or task force for project implementation. Donor willingness to fund operations and maintenance, and not only infrastructure, could help ensure sustained operations of existing and future water and wastewater plants.
- Reconsider immediate funding cuts to humanitarian causes in Gaza to include a phased and more structured withdrawal of support from UNRWA.
- Increase funds for public health risk mitigation initiatives.
- Relax restrictions on access and movement of goods. Israel and Egypt need to weigh their legitimate security concerns against Gaza's humanitarian needs and the real risk of a public health crisis spilling across Gaza's borders and into Israeli and Egyptian territory. While Israel committed to allow the entrance of materials needed for water, wastewater, and WASH projects in Gaza, the process is cumbersome and delays implementation. A strong level of international political engagement could guarantee that Israel's commitment to support WASH projects will be translated into efficient and rapid processing of demands and authorize the entry of required dual-use materials for these projects.

- Identify trusted third parties to mediate intra-Palestinian disputes over issues like ongoing payments for water and electricity.
- Form international coalitions to address issues of regional concern.
- Address development needs alongside humanitarian relief to alleviate Gaza's dependence on international assistance and help it become more self-sufficient.

Conclusion

While the solutions to Gaza's electricity, water, and public health problems are technical in nature, the reality is that Gaza's access to energy, water, and financial resources depends largely on whether Hamas, the PA, Israel, and Egypt can reconcile their political differences and whether the international community can successfully navigate these political complexities. Even though the international community has repeatedly pledged donations for large-scale energy and water projects in Gaza, follow-through on these commitments has been lacking. In addition, given the complex political dynamic between the different stakeholders in the region, international donors are reluctant to continue funding major projects in Gaza. Some of the proposed solutions require funding of operations and maintenance or investment on the Israeli side (e.g., the 161kV line), which donors are not willing to fund. These solutions have been deterred by the intra-Palestinian rivalry, continued limitations of access and movement imposed by Israel and Egypt, and lack of proper governance in the energy and water sectors. Addressing these issues is therefore necessary to bring long-term and systemic changes to Gaza's water and energy sectors, which will in turn help improve public health there. At the same time, efforts to cope (even partially) with the political challenges should be accompanied by short-term stabilization and risk mitigation measures that can be advanced immediately to prevent a large-scale public health crisis.

Acknowledgments

The authors thank our formal peer reviewers, including RAND Corporation colleagues Michelle Miro, hydrologist and associate engineer; and Laura Faherty, associate physician policy researcher. Celine Touboul, deputy director general and senior researcher of the Economic Cooperation Foundation, also provided valuable feedback on this report. We further thank the many individuals and institutions who helped enhance our understating of the technical and political complexities of Gaza, including researchers at the Institute for National Security Studies (INSS); experts at the United Nations, the World Health Organization, and the Quartet; Israeli and Palestinian officials; and others, many of whom chose to remain anonymous. We also thank the RAND Center for Middle East Public Policy, its director, Dalia Dassa Kaye, and its advisory board for supporting and funding this project.

Abbreviations

CMWU	Coastal Municipalities Water Utility
GEDCO	Gaza Electricity Distribution Company
GPP	Gaza Power Plant
GVC	Gruppo di Volontariato Civile
INSS	Institute for National Security Studies
KAP	knowledge, attitudes, and practices
KFW	German Development Bank
mcm	million cubic meters
MECIDS	Middle East Consortium on Infectious Disease Surveillance
MoEHE	Ministry of Education and Higher Education
MICS	Multiple Indicator Cluster Survey
MoU	memorandum of understanding
MW	megawatts
NGEST	North Gaza Emergency Sewage Treatment
NGO	nongovernmental organization
NO_2	nitrite
NO_3	nitrate
OCHA	United Nations Office for the Coordination of Humanitarian Affairs
PA	Palestinian Authority

POU	point-of-use
PWA	Palestinian Water Authority
STLV	Short-Term Low-Volume
UAE	United Arab Emirates
UN	United Nations
UNHCR	United Nations High Commissioner for Refugees
UNICEF	United Nations Children's Fund
UNRWA	United Nations Relief and Works Agency
UNSCO	Office of the United Nations Special Coordinator for the Middle East Peace Process
WASH	water, sanitation, and hygiene
WHO	World Health Organization
WWTP	wastewater treatment plant

CHAPTER ONE

Introduction

In Gaza, one crisis is playing out in public while another happens behind the scenes. After dozens of Palestinians died and hundreds were wounded in clashes with the Israeli military in a series of demonstrations at the border that began on March 30, 2018,[1] Palestinians in Gaza began flying kites with flammable material and explosive balloons into Israel on a daily basis, leading to arsons associated with damage to crops and forests of millions of dollars.[2] Israel has accused Hamas of these attacks and retaliated by striking Hamas positions and cells.[3] The conflict has drawn renewed attention to Gaza, especially as Israel and Hamas have been working behind the scenes to agree to a ceasefire.[4] But it masks an emergency that affects far more Gaza residents and has the potential to spread beyond its borders: Gaza has a water and sanitation crisis of epic proportions.

Both the security and water crises are driven by similar causes: governance failure; a power struggle between the rival Palestinian factions (Hamas, the de facto government of Gaza, and the Fatah-led Palestinian Authority [PA], based in the West Bank); high population

---

[1] Beverley Milton-Edwards, "Gaza Protests Highlight Humanitarian Crisis and Lack of Political Progress to Peace," Brookings Institution, April 5, 2018.

[2] Almog Ben Zikri, "Flammable Kites from Gaza Set Israeli Fields and Forests Ablaze," *Haaretz*, May 23, 2018.

[3] Nikki Guttman, "IDF Photos Prove Hamas Is Behind Gaza Kite Terrorism," *Israel Hayom*, June 26, 2018.

[4] "Report: Israel-Hamas Ceasefire Deal Nears Completion," Tazpit Press Service, August 24, 2018.

density; three wars between Hamas and Israel in five years (2009 to 2014); and severe restrictions on imports, exports, and travel to and from Gaza. All these factors have brought Gaza to the brink of collapse. Add aging infrastructure to this mix, and the result is a water and sanitation emergency that affects public health inside and outside Gaza—as illustrated by the death in 2017 of a five-year-old boy after swimming in sewage-contaminated seawater.[5]

As this report shows, Gaza's water issue is twofold—a shortage of potable water combined with lack of wastewater sanitation. The first part of this problem is a lack of access to plentiful and safe water for drinking, cooking, and personal and domestic hygiene, which is a serious threat to public health. The second issue is ineffective sanitation, which results in more than 108,000 cubic meters of untreated sewage—equivalent to 43 Olympic-size swimming pools—flowing daily from Gaza into the Mediterranean Sea,[6] creating extreme public health security risks in Gaza and in neighboring Israel and Egypt. In addition, partially treated wastewater infiltrates into the groundwater in North Gaza.[7]

Even though the water and sanitation crisis is not a new phenomenon in Gaza—the strip of coastal land could be described as in a chronic state of water emergency—a confluence of negative developments has exacerbated the situation and intensified the associated health risks. First is the continued depletion of the coastal aquifer, Gaza's only source of freshwater, which is not sufficient to meet the needs of its approximately 2 million Palestinian residents. Decades of overpumping, combined with the seepage of wastewater and agrochemicals and seawater intrusion, have brought the aquifer to a possibly irrecoverable state.[8] As a result, some 97 percent of the aquifer's ground-

---

[5] Adel Zaanoun, "Death of Gazan Boy Puts Spotlight on Polluted Water," *Times of Israel*, August 26, 2017.

[6] United Nations (UN), *Gaza Ten Years Later*, July 2017b.

[7] Palestinian Water Authority (PWA) official, email exchange with authors, April 12, 2018.

[8] "Gaza in 2020: A Liveable Place?" press release, United Nations Relief and Works Agency for Palestine Refugees in the Near East, August 28, 2012.

water is already unfit for human consumption, according to World Health Organization (WHO) water quality standards.[9] The yield of the aquifer is estimated at 55 to 60 million cubic meters (mcm) per year, but total water demand in Gaza is 180 mcm per year.[10] Demand for scarce potable water sources in Gaza is only going to rise with an expected population growth of over 3.2 percent per year; household water demand is expected to increase from 103 mcm in 2015 to 140 mcm in 2035.[11] Figure 1.1 illustrates water scarcity.

Moreover, recurring conflict with Israel has severely damaged the water, sanitation, and hygiene (WASH) infrastructure in Gaza.

Figure 1.1
Potable Water Sources Are Scarce in Gaza

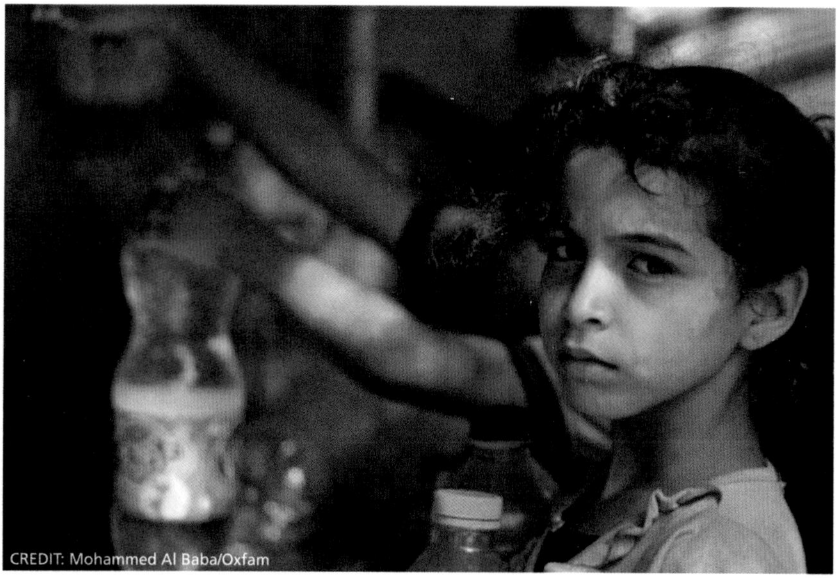

Children in Rafah collect water from one of the working public taps. Unaltered image licensed through Creative Commons: https://creativecommons.org/licenses/by-sa/4.0/legalcode

9 "Report: 97% of Gaza's Drinking Water at Sewer Quality," JNi.Media, January 21, 2018.

10 European Commission, "Giving Gaza Hope: Gaza Central Desalination Plant Providing Water to 2 Million People," fact sheet, undated.

11 European Commission, undated.

For example, a Palestinian official report assessed the damage of the 2014 Israeli Operation Protective Edge to WASH infrastructure at $34 million. This includes damage to groundwater wells, water reservoirs, wastewater treatment plants (WWTPs), collection networks and pumping stations, desalination plants, and other facilities.[12] Despite international pledges to fund the reconstruction of houses and infrastructure destroyed in the war, as of March 2018, a funding gap of $244 million remained, including $20 million for energy infrastructure and $11 million for water infrastructure.[13] The U.S. decision to cut $200 million in bilateral aid to the Palestinians, including for water and humanitarian projects in the West Bank and Gaza, will exacerbate funding shortages.[14]

Furthermore, severe restrictions on access and movement imposed by Israel and Egypt have hindered post-conflict repair and rebuilding. Israel tightly restricts the importation of a list of dual-use items that could be used for both civilian and military purposes, for instance. This list includes 70 percent of the technical equipment needed for the WASH sector, such as pumps and chemicals for water purification. In response to months of attacks from Gaza using fire kites and balloons mounted with incendiary devices, Israel in July 2018 temporarily shut down Kerem Shalom, the main crossing of goods into Gaza, to all imports and exports except for food, medicine, and "humanitarian equipment." This decision included a temporary halt on importation of fuel and gas.[15] While Israel has since then reopened the crossing, access and movement have remained severely restricted. As of July 2018, Egypt has kept Rafah, its only border crossing with Gaza, mostly

---

12 Coastal Municipalities Water Utility (CMWU), *Damages Assessment Report, Water and Wastewater Infrastructure (Gaza Strip; July 7–August 14, 2014)*, August 2014.

13 Office of the United Nations Special Coordinator for the Middle East Peace Process (UNSCO), *Report to the Ad Hoc Liaison Committee*, Brussels: United Nations, March 20, 2018.

14 Gardiner Harris, "Trump Administration Cuts More Than $200 Million in Aid for Palestinians," *New York Times*, August 24, 2018.

15 "Israel Cuts Gas, Fuel to Gaza as Egypt Shuts Rafah Gate," *Daily Sabah*, July 17, 2018.

closed since 2014, citing security concerns.[16] In May 2018, Egypt kept Rafah open for the whole month of Ramadan,[17] but in July 2018 it announced that it would close the crossing "indefinitely."[18]

The state of the WASH sector is linked directly to a chronic energy shortage in Gaza. As will be explained in Chapter Two, Gaza's residents normally receive their electricity supply from three sources: Israel, Egypt, and domestic power generation—none of which, as of 2018, is reliable. The electricity deficit crisis has worsened since mid-2017 due to an intra-Palestinian dispute between the PA and Hamas over payments for the electricity imported from Israel. Although this issue was addressed, the PA has imposed requirements that have limited other sources of supply, including a new tax on imported fuel amounting to 100 percent of refined fuel prices, leading to a decline in fuel purchases for Gaza's only internal source of power: the Gaza Power Plant (GPP).[19] Lack of diesel fuel, for example, caused a temporary shutdown of the GPP in February 2018. All in all, as of June 2018, Gaza's residents receive power for only four hours at a time, followed by 16 hours of blackout.[20]

The shortage of electricity and fuel to operate water and wastewater treatment facilities has further reduced Gaza's already limited access to clean water and sanitation solutions. Between the fall of 2016 and the summer of 2017, 186 facilities providing health, water and sanitation, and solid waste collection services were shut down due to power shortages.[21] In February 2018, municipalities in Gaza announced that, due to the severe energy and funding crises, they would be cutting their services in half. Insufficient electricity for wastewater treatment

---

[16] "Egypt Opens Border with Gaza Temporarily," *The National*, February 21, 2018.

[17] "Egypt Opens Gaza's Rafah Crossing for Ramadan," Associated Press, May 18, 2018.

[18] "Israel Cuts Gas, Fuel to Gaza as Egypt Shuts Rafah Gate," 2018.

[19] Oren Liebermann and Talal Abu Rahma, "Gaza Crippled by Electricity Crisis as Power Plant Runs out of Fuel," CNN, April 17, 2017.

[20] Jack Khoury, "Gaza on 4 Hours of Power a Day After Sole Electric Firm Shuts Down," *Haaretz*, February 22, 2018.

[21] UN Office for the Coordination of Humanitarian Affairs (OCHA), "The Humanitarian Impact of the Internal Palestinian Divide on the Gaza Strip," fact sheet, June 23, 2017a.

has also led to beach closures where untreated sewage flows directly into the sea.[22]

The financial crisis in Gaza and difficulties in implementing large-scale projects have contributed to the steady deterioration of the energy and WASH sectors, exacerbating health risks not only in Gaza, but also in neighboring Israel and Egypt. The U.S. decision to cut $300 million in funding to the UN Relief and Works Agency (UNRWA), the UN fund that supports Palestinian refugees, could further worsen the situation.[23] UNRWA supports the WASH sector and provides public health services in Gaza: Specifically, it operates 21 primary health clinics, employs more than 1,000 staff in the WASH sector (out of a total UNRWA staff of 13,000 in Gaza),[24] serves more than 4 million annual patient visits, and runs schools where some WASH educational programs are taught.[25] These services are critical, as Gaza's hospitals are becoming increasingly inoperable.[26]

While the solutions to Gaza's electricity, water, and public health problems are technical in nature, they depend on whether Hamas, the PA, Israel, Egypt, and the international community can reconcile their political differences. Lessons since Hamas violently took control over Gaza in 2007 indicate that politics often trump public health or humanitarian considerations. As stakeholders recognize the impact of these political challenges and seek to overcome the difficulties in addressing them, it is important that they enact steps that would help stabilize Gaza and prevent a humanitarian crisis that could also affect Israel, Egypt, and other countries in the region.

---

22 "Municipal Services in Gaza Reduced by 50%," *Middle East Monitor*, February 22, 2018.

23 In January 2018, the United States announced a decision to contribute only $60 million to UNRWA's 2018 budget, as compared with a total contribution exceeding $353 million for 2017 for the regular budget and emergency appeals for the West Bank and Gaza and for Syria (Karen DeYoung, Ruth Eglash, and Hazem Balousha, "U.S. Ends Aid to United Nations Agency Supporting Palestinian Refugees," *Washington Post*, August 31, 2018).

24 Nidal al-Mughrabi, "UN Employees in Gaza Demonstrate Against U.S. Aid Cut," Reuters, January 28, 2018b.

25 UNRWA, "Occupied Palestinian Territory Emergency Appeal 2018," January 30, 2018.

26 Ahmad Abu Amer, "Unpaid Gaza Employees Lash out at Qatari Ambassador," *Al-Monitor*, February 26, 2018.

This report explains Gaza's dual water and sanitation problem, discusses the linkages between Gaza's energy and water crises and the risks to public health, and evaluates policy options for mitigating the different issues. The analysis draws on a variety of sources, including reports from government and international aid organizations, such as the UN, the Office of the Quartet (an organization that includes the United Nations, United States, European Union, and Russia), the World Bank, WHO, and others; policy papers by think tanks and research institutes; hundreds of media and news reports; and off-the-record semistructured and open-ended conversations with dozens of experts from the UN, WHO, nongovernmental organizations (NGOs) and current and former Israeli, Palestinian, and U.S. government officials. While these sources vary in their levels of detail and credibility, journalistic accounts and interviews are necessary in lieu of empirical literature, which has lagged behind developments on the ground. These sources are also important given the challenge of collecting public health data in Gaza[27]—especially barriers to research teams wishing to visit Gaza and collect data in person.

In the remainder of this report, we begin by presenting a snapshot of Gaza's limited electricity, poor domestic water supply, and state of wastewater sanitation. Subsequently, we describe water-related risks to public health in Gaza, particularly those of inadequate water quality due to chemical and biological contamination and those resulting from inadequate water quantity. Further, we explore the health risks that Gaza's water problems could pose for Israel and Egypt. We conclude by evaluating various steps to ameliorate the water and sanitation crisis and reduce the likelihood of a significant public health disaster in Gaza and its neighbors, taking into account the significant political constraints.

---

27 Rasha Khatib, Rita Giacaman, Umaiyeh Khammash, and Salim Yusuf, "Challenges to Conducting Epidemiology Research in Chronic Conflict Areas: Examples from PURE-Palestine," *Conflict and Health*, Vol. 10, No. 1, 2016, p. 33.

CHAPTER TWO

Water and Wastewater Services in Gaza

Though Gaza encompasses only a 365-square-kilometer area, population estimates suggest that there are between 1.85 million and 2 million people currently inhabiting the small strip of land, making it one of the most dense population centers in the world.[1] If current trends continue, the UN projects that number will reach 3.1 million by 2030 and 4.7 million by 2050, creating untenable demands on already insufficient infrastructure and resources.[2] Perhaps nowhere is this strain more evident than in the water sector. Gaza's water infrastructure is degraded and was designed at a capacity that is unable to support the growing population. In addition, the quality and quantity of water produced by treatment plants is insufficient for the requirements of populated urban centers. Furthermore, Gaza's wastewater infrastructure is also in disrepair, and insufficient electrical power supply leaves large parts of the population with no wastewater services. The 2014 conflict between Israel and Hamas and its aftermath seriously degraded the already limited capacity, and ongoing embargoes on construction material and other supplies have diminished the ability to make necessary repairs, creating a water and wastewater emergency in Gaza.

Inadequate infrastructure is only one component of the current water emergencies; the other is the overwhelming dependence on a scarce and largely unsafe water supply that is nevertheless used by inhab-

---

1 Palestinian Central Bureau of Statistics, "Palestinians' Population Status in the Palestine, 2016 (Arabic only)," State of Palestine, 2016.

2 "Population Growth in Occupied Palestinian Territory to Drive Demand for Housing, Services—UN," press release, UN News Center, December 21, 2016.

itants to wash, cook, and drink. Specifically, Gaza's single coastal aquifer accounts for 95 percent of available freshwater, and this source is being rapidly depleted and suffers from heightening seawater intrusion. Additionally, the CMWU supplies domestic water only to residents who can afford the steep cost of water delivery services. A further number of residents rely on unregulated brackish water desalination plants (BWDPs) that provide only part-time service. A small fraction of the population purchases bottled water for home use at an exorbitant cost. This chapter will discuss the primary sources of water available to residents in Gaza, the advantages and limitations associated with each source, and the difficulties of using current water and wastewater conveyance and treatment infrastructure given ongoing technical and electrical supply challenges.

Gaza's Water Supply: Limited in Both Quantity and Quality—and Unaffordable

The Coastal Aquifer

The coastal aquifer that accounts for 95 percent of available freshwater in Gaza extends from the town of Binyamina, south of Haifa in the northern part of Israel, to the Sinai Desert in Egypt to the south (Figure 2.1). In total, the aquifer encompasses an area of 18,370 square kilometers, of which 71 percent is in Egypt, 27 percent in Israel, and the final 2 percent in the State of Palestine, primarily in Gaza. While only 2 percent of the entire groundwater basin is accessible from Gaza, the population living in that area has historically been heavily dependent on it. As shown in Figure 2.1, the groundwater level is highest and above sea level in places extending away from the Gaza boundary and is at or below sea level in population centers in Rafah, Khan Yunis, and Gaza City, where the aquifer has been heavily drawn down to support water demand. The aquifer extends across three different territories, and groundwater extractions are divided among the territories—approximately 66 percent from Israel, 23 percent from Gaza, and 11 percent from Egypt.[3]

---

[3] *Inventory of Shared Water Resources in Western Asia*, Beirut, Lebanon: UN Economic and Social Commission for Western Asia and German Federal Institute for Geosciences and Natural Resources, 2013.

Figure 2.1
Groundwater Level in the Coastal Aquifer (2004–2005 Data)

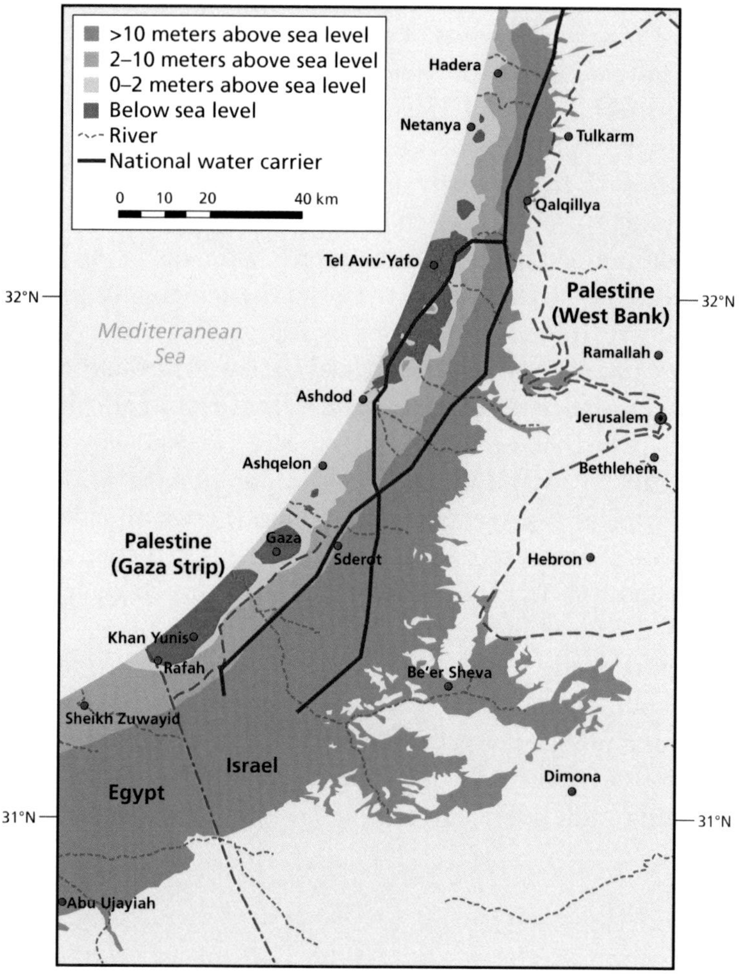

SOURCE: *Inventory of Shared Water Resources in Western Asia*, 2013.

Through the late 1990s, the aquifer's available fresh water supplied most of Gaza's residents with drinkable tap water. But since then, water demand has increased to the point that groundwater is no longer naturally replenished at a rate that can meet demand.[4] Groundwater in the coastal aquifer typically recharges from several sources, predominant among them rainfall infiltration, at the rate of 50 to 60 mcm annually. However, Palestinian extraction of groundwater currently hovers around 160 mcm per year, which is nearly three times the annual recharge rate.[5] Even with a reduced extraction rate, the PWA estimates that 91 mcm is the minimum required to meet domestic supply, which is still nearly double the average recharge rate in the coastal aquifer.[6]

In addition to the diminishing supply, water quality in the coastal aquifer continues to decline. As the groundwater level drops below sea level, fresh water quality is degraded by seawater intrusion. At the same time, untreated or insufficiently treated wastewater from nearby population centers and refugee camps and runoff from agricultural areas have all increased the aquifer's salinity to levels beyond what the WHO considers safe for potable water.[7] Furthermore, runoff from sewage and farmland irrigation brings nitrate and chloride contamination into the aquifer, which can pose significant health risks if present at elevated levels. The public health risks associated with this chemical contamination are discussed in detail in the next chapter.

Because water from the coastal aquifer is both increasingly depleted and polluted, it is no longer the primary source for drinking water for the millions of people living in Gaza. Instead, residents primarily use water taken directly from the aquifer for personal hygiene and cleaning while relying on other sources for drinking and cooking.[8]

---

4 "Water Situation Alarming in Gaza," World Bank, November 22, 2016.

5 "Gaza in 2020: A Liveable Place?" 2012.

6 PWA, "Terms of Reference for the Associated Works for Gaza Desalination Project," April 2014.

7 *Inventory of Shared Water Resources in Western Asia*, 2013.

8 Oded Eran, Gidon Bromberg, and Michal Milner, *The Water, Sanitation, and Energy Crises in Gaza: Humanitarian, Environmental and Geopolitical Implications with Recommendations for Immediate Measures*, Tel Aviv: EcoPeace Middle East, August 11, 2014.

Other Sources of Supply

Purchased, imported water has been a part of Gaza's supply mix for the past several decades. Israel's National Water Company, Mekorot, started selling potable water to Gaza in 1980. But this quantity has always represented only a small fraction of Gaza's total water demand. In March 2015, faced with increasing risks connected to Gaza's water crisis, Israel committed to doubling the amount of potable water sold, from 5 to 10 mcm per year.[9] However, due to limited storage capacity, Israel provided only 8 mcm until early 2017, when the German Development Bank (KFW) completed the refurbishment of the Al Muntar reservoir in Gaza City.[10]

In July 2017, the PA and Israel reached, in principle, a new water sale agreement under which the PA would be able to buy an additional 33 mcm of potable water per year from Israel, of which 10 mcm would be delivered to Gaza.[11] Based on the capacity of the existing pipelines, Israel could immediately provide the first 5 mcm of water. Further investments, however, are needed to build a new pipeline connecting Israel to Gaza to supply the remaining 5 mcm. As of August 2018, the agreement has not been finalized.[12] Once it is fully implemented, Gaza will purchase a total of 20 mcm per year. The imported water could be blended with groundwater to make roughly 40 mcm of potable water available. Though an increase from previous agreements, this amount is still insufficient to meet demand in Gaza.

Water Treatment, Storage, and Distribution

The 2014 Multiple Indicator Cluster Survey (MICS) of Gaza and the West Bank identified tube-wells or bore holes, protected wells, protected

---

[9] In 1995, as part of the interim agreement between Israel and the Palestine Liberation Organization, Israel committed to selling Gaza 5 mcm of water annually.

[10] Gidon Bromberg, Giulia Giordano, Oded Eran, and Omri Elad, "Gaza on the Edge: The Water and Energy Crisis in Gaza," Ecopeace Middle East and Institute for National Security Studies (INSS), May 2018.

[11] Ahmad Melhem, "Israeli-Palestinian Water Pact Raises Hopes, Suspicions," *Al-Monitor*, July 25, 2017.

[12] Conversation with official at the Office of the Quartet, Jerusalem, July 13, 2018.

springs, rainwater collection, and bottled water as forms of improved drinking-water sources.[13] An improved water source, as defined by the WHO/United Nations Children's Fund (UNICEF) Joint Monitoring Programme for Water Supply and Sanitation, is that which, "by nature of its construction and when properly used, adequately protects the source from outside contamination, particularly fecal matter."[14]

While the West Bank also suffers water shortages and sanitation issues, water supply and quality are substantially better there than in Gaza. The survey found that while 88.9 percent of household respondents in the West Bank had access to some form of improved drinking water, only 10.1 percent of households in Gaza benefited from the same access.[15] See Figure 2.2 for a comparison of household drinking-water sources in Gaza and the West Bank in 2014. Instead of using improved drinking sources, the large majority of households in Gaza get their water from water trucks, carts, or public filling points (Figure 2.2 and Figure 2.3).[16]

Figure 2.3 presents an updated picture of household water sources in Gaza. It describes the distribution of household drinking water sources in 2017, prior to implementation of the water sales agreement between Israel and the PA.[17] The chronic shortage of safe water has led Gaza's residents to increasingly depend on small-scale desalination of brackish water conducted by private vendors. Figures 2.2 and 2.3 also show that the amount of drinking water available in homes

---

13 "West Bank and Gaza—Multiple Indicator Cluster Survey 2014," World Bank, 2014. Hereafter, this survey will be cited as "MICS, 2014."

14 WHO/UNICEF Joint Monitoring Programme, "Improved and Unimproved Water Sources and Sanitation Facilities," undated.

15 WHO/UNICEF Joint Monitoring Programme, undated, p. 81.

16 PWA, Gruppo di Volontariato Civile (GVC) Italia, and UNICEF, "Water, Sanitation and Hygiene Assessment at the Household Level in the Gaza Strip," 2017.

17 The data sources for Figure 2.2 and Figure 2.3 do not necessarily align and show a large variation in the percentage accessing water from tanker trucks. This could be explained by differences in what was counted as a "tanker truck" versus "cart" in the MICS survey or other differences in how each category was described. The discrepancy could also be due to differing samples (nationally representative although different in size) from different periods (2014 versus 2017).

Figure 2.2
Household Drinking Water Sources by Percentage in Gaza Versus the West Bank (2014)

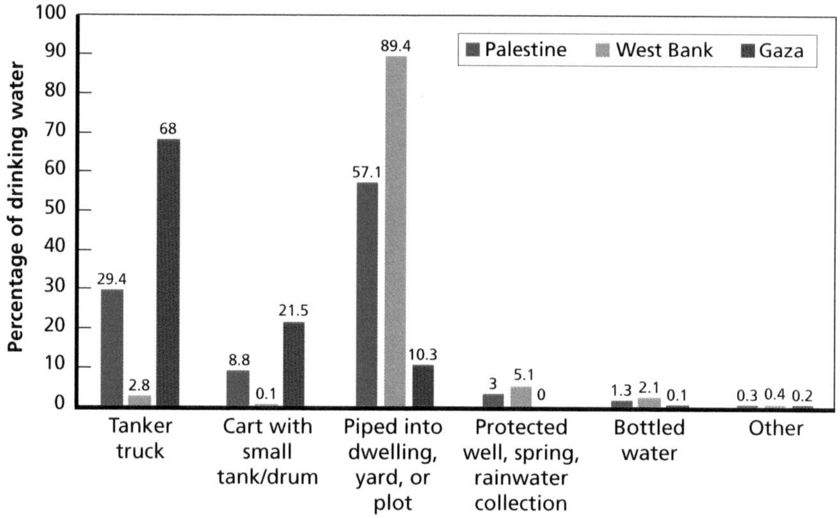

SOURCE: MICS, 2014.

Figure 2.3
Household Drinking-Water Sources in Gaza by Percentage (2017)

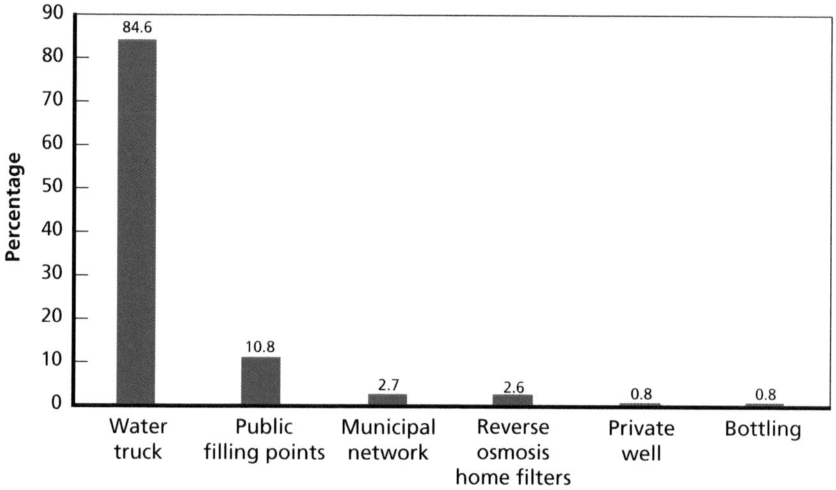

SOURCE: PWA, GVC, and UNICEF, 2017.

via municipal supply, private wells, or home reverse osmosis treatment appears to have declined (6.1 percent in 2017).

Per a 2016 report, nine in ten people in Gaza drink desalinated water produced by 154 public and private desalination plants, only 48 of which are licensed and monitored.[18] Even if these small desalination plants reduce salinity, they do not necessarily effectively remove other pollutants. In addition, the small desalination plants are currently functioning at 15 percent of their capacity due to insufficient power supply.[19] As of January 2017, two large public desalination plants were operating in Gaza, and there have been ongoing efforts supported by international funding to increase desalination capacity.[20] These large desalination plants provide only 4 percent of drinking water, however, because of the limited electricity supply available, as we will discuss later.[21] The PWA, with the support of international donors, has made progress toward the construction of a Gaza Central Desalination Program, which will provide 55 mcm of potable water per year after completion of its initial phase and by 2023 help meet the expected demand of 139 mcm. As of late March 2018, however, international funding to begin construction is some $230 million short. This plant will also require a sustained power supply.[22]

Scarcity has made water very expensive in Gaza, despite its low quality and inconsistent supply. UN standards for affordable water state that the cost of water should not exceed 3 percent of household income.[23] However, according to a survey from 2010, some residents of

---

18 Emergency Water, Sanitation, and Hygiene Group, "Life Under Blockade: 86% of Projects Necessary to Develop the Ravaged WASH Sector in Gaza Remain at Risk," press release, March 22, 2016.

19 Emergency Water, Sanitation, and Hygiene Group, 2016.

20 "Water Situation Alarming in Gaza," 2016.

21 "Water Situation Alarming in Gaza," 2016.

22 Office of the Quartet, *Report to the Ad Hoc Liaison Committee*, Brussels, March 20, 2018.

23 UN, "Global Issues: Water," fact sheet, undated.

Gaza spend as much as a third of their income on water, and 83 percent of households reported relying mainly on private vendors.[24]

Other families without the capacity to pay for private water vendors rely on unregulated wells.[25] Nonpayment for water is rampant at 57 percent of all households, of which 87 percent do not pay because of economic circumstances or lack of social responsibility.[26]

One way to ameliorate low rates of access to improved drinking water sources is to use safe water treatment practices, including boiling water before drinking it, using a water filter at the point of use, adding bleach or chlorine to the water, or allowing the water to stand and settle before use. The 2014 MICS survey found, however, that nearly 94 percent of households in Gaza reported using no water treatment method on unimproved drinking water.[27] This highlights an area for potential improvement: educating households on the importance of enacting such practices to improve the quality of water they consume. Insufficient access to safe water also limits personal hygiene (e.g., for handwashing or bathing) and domestic hygiene (e.g., for cleaning food, utensils, floors). Together, inadequate hygiene, combined with an overreliance on unimproved water, creates ideal conditions for disease transmission.

Given the elevated health risks from unsafe drinking water to children and youth, it is relevant to present data on water availability in schools (Figure 2.4). According to a survey of schools in the Palestinian Territories conducted in 2015–2016, the main source of water in Gaza's schools is tank truck deliveries from the Palestinian Ministry of Education and Higher Education (MoEHE) and UNICEF, a private vendor, or from other humanitarian aid organizations. That is in contrast to most schools (93 percent) in the West Bank, for which the main source of water is the public network.

---

[24] MICS, 2014.

[25] Maayan Niezna, *Hand on the Switch: Who's Responsible for Gaza's Infrastructure Crisis?* Tel Aviv–Jaffa, Israel: Gisha—Legal Center for Freedom of Movement, January 2017.

[26] PWA, GVC Italia, and UNICEF, 2017, p. 51.

[27] MICS, 2014, p. 84.

Figure 2.4
Water Sources and Treatment in Schools in Gaza Compared with the West Bank

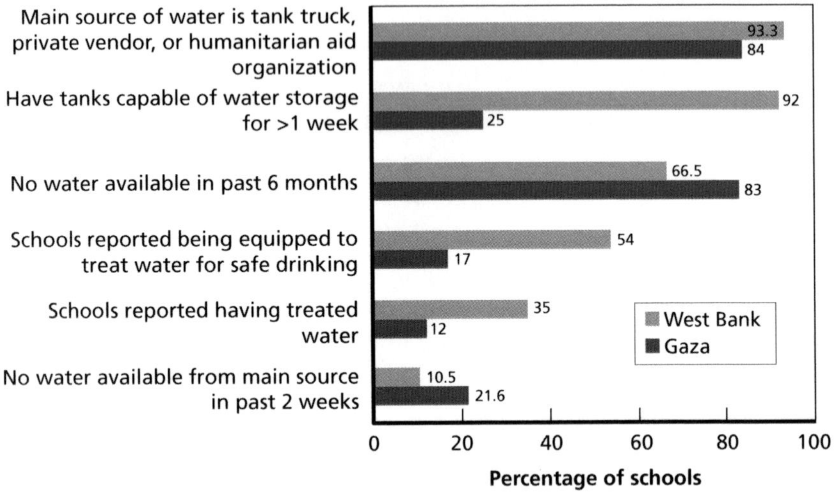

SOURCE: MoEHE, UNICEF in the State of Palestine, and Alpha International, "Water, Sanitation and Hygiene in Schools; Knowledge, Attitudes and Practices Survey: 2015–2016," December 2016.

Furthermore, only 12 percent of surveyed Gaza schools reported treating their water (compared with 35 percent of West Bank schools). Here, *treatment* primarily refers to adding chlorine, using a water filter, letting the water sit and settle, and boiling. However, 83 percent of schools in Gaza reported that they are not adequately equipped to treat water for safe drinking (compared with 46 percent of schools in the West Bank). The survey took place in 2015–2016, before the deterioration in the humanitarian situation of 2017, so water safety in Gaza schools may have further declined as of the writing of this report in summer 2018.

Sewage Treatment Is Only Partially Operational

More than a quarter of Gaza residents live in areas without adequate sanitary sewage infrastructure.[28] In 2011, the sanitary sewage network covered only two-thirds of Gaza's population and was then in a state of disrepair. The remaining third used cesspits and open drains to dispose of their wastewater. The lack of adequate wastewater sanitation stems from two main causes: delays in completion of three wastewater treatment facilities, and the lack of a reliable energy supply to operate such plants.

This problem is not new. In the past, periodic cuts to the energy supply, often following direct Israel-Hamas confrontations, have led to outages or malfunctions in the sanitation systems. In 2006, cuts to the fuel supply affected the operations of wastewater pumping stations, as well as wastewater treatment.

Today, the CMWU has only limited available power, which it uses to operate 55 sewage pumping stations and five partially operational WWTPs.[29] When the plants cannot treat incoming wastewater, it is instead discharged into the Mediterranean. Currently, some 108,000 cubic meters of untreated or poorly treated sewage are discharged into the sea every day.[30] This pollution, according to reports, was the reason for the death of the five-year-old boy in July 2017[31] and for shutting down the Ashkelon desalination plant in 2016.[32] If present trends continue, the amount of sewage dumped into Gaza's sea might increase to 120,000 cubic meters per day.[33]

In early 2018, the long-awaited Northern Gaza Emergency Sewage Treatment (NGEST) facility became operational. The facility

---

28 Emergency Water, Sanitation, and Hygiene Group, "Water and Sanitation in Palestine," fact sheet, 2017.

29 UN, 2017b.

30 See comments by Eilon Adar of Ben-Gurion University in Shlomi Eldar, "Gaza's Ticking Sewage Bomb," *Al-Monitor*, June 16, 2017.

31 Zaanoun, 2017.

32 Yisrael Price, "Gaza Sewage Threatens Israel's Water Supply," *Hamodia*, March 21, 2016.

33 UN, 2017b.

is designed to provide a sustainable wastewater management solution for 400,000 residents of northern Gaza communities.[34] However, NGEST still faces two key issues. First, there is a $16.8 million funding gap to cover operations and maintenance costs.[35] This is not a large sum relative to the cost of construction of the plant (some $100 million),[36] but while donors are willing to fund infrastructure, they are reluctant to pay for operations and maintenance; these are recurring costs that need a sustainable solution.[37] The PWA and other stakeholders need to identify sources of support to finance the cost of NGEST's operation and delegate the operations and maintenance to the CMWU. The second issue is that NGEST needs a constant power supply to operate in a sustainable manner.[38] This example illustrates one of the central challenges to consistent water and wastewater service provision—limited availability of electricity, as discussed in the next section.

Energy Scarcity Complicates Water and Wastewater Treatment

Gaza's Energy Crisis

Gaza's water problems are directly linked to a prolonged energy crisis. Gaza has not had a regular electricity supply in over a decade, and until 2017 households, on average, had power for 12 to 16 hours per day. Gaza's residents have normally received their electricity supply from three unreliable sources: imports from Israel, imports from Egypt, and domestic power generation. While as of March 2018, electricity demand in Gaza was 473 to 496 megawatts (MW) per day, supply

---

[34] Office of the Quartet, 2018.

[35] Office of the Quartet, 2018. The Office of the Quartet indicated that "donors are encouraged to meet the remaining shortfall" in funding, yet as of summer 2018, the funding gap remains.

[36] "Northern Gaza Emergency Sewage Treatment (NGEST) Project," fact sheet, World Bank, July 15, 2018.

[37] Conversation with official at the Office of the Quartet, Jerusalem, July 13, 2018.

[38] Phone conversation with UN officials based in Jerusalem, March 4, 2018.

amounted to only 164 MW per day.[39] Until 2017, Gaza's electricity grid had provided about 208 MW per day—slightly more than in 2018 but still insufficient.[40] More than half of this power, 120 MW per day, is sold and supplied by Israel through ten medium-voltage lines. When fuel is imported and available, an additional 60 MW are produced by the GPP, which is less than half its capacity, and another 20 to 30 MW have been sold by Egypt.[41]

The GPP fuel supply is inconsistent and expensive. In 2017, the PA imposed a new tax on fuel, amounting to 100 percent of refined fuel prices, leading to a decline in fuel purchases for the plant.[42] The GPP was shut down in April 2017 due to these price increases, cutting Gaza's electricity supply by roughly another 30 percent.[43] Making matters worse, Egypt's power lines into Gaza became nonoperational, cutting electricity supply from Egypt to zero.[44] By mid-2017, this left Gaza dependent on the 120 MW per day imported from Israel.

Electricity imports from Israel, however, have also proven unreliable due to ongoing political disputes. Traditionally, the PA has paid for Gaza's electricity imports from both Israel and Egypt. The cost of Israeli imported electricity is deducted from the revenue that Israel collects on imported goods and transfers to the PA.[45] In June 2017, the PA announced that it would cut back its payments for power from Israel for Gaza by $12 million per month and requested that Israel correspondingly reduce power supply to Gaza from 120 MW to 70 MW per day. The PA conditioned its resumption of electric power purchases on Hamas transferring over the fees and taxes it collects from Gaza's resi-

---

[39] Office of the Quartet, 2018.

[40] UN, "Humanitarian Impact of the Gaza Electricity Crisis," May 2017a.

[41] UN, 2017a.

[42] Liebermann and Abu Rahma, 2017.

[43] Bromberg et al., 2017.

[44] Conversation with officials at the UN, Jerusalem, July 13, 2018.

[45] Diana B. Greenwald, "Who Is Responsible for Solving Gaza's Massive Electricity Crisis?" *Washington Post*, February 5, 2018.

dents. The dispute left residents of Gaza with three hours of electricity per day for seven months.[46]

As a result of Egyptian mediation aimed at reconciling the two sides and bringing the PA back to Gaza to reassume its governance role, the PA resumed full electricity payments to Israel in January 2018. Nevertheless, as of July 2018, reconciliation continues to be an unmet goal, hindering further improvements to Gaza's electricity supply. Specifically, as the PA enabled the restoration of power supply from Israel, it required Gaza Electricity Distribution Company (GEDCO), the local power utility, to contribute 10 million Israeli shekels (about $3 million) toward the purchase of Israeli electricity.[47] GEDCO promised to collect payments from consumers, and Israel restored the power supply. Faced with this new expenditure and with limited available funds, GEDCO was forced to reduce fuel purchases for the GPP.[48] In the period between January 22 and March 20, 2018, the GPP reduced production substantially, producing at most 25 MW of electricity per day.[49] In addition, it has occasionally shut down completely due to lack of fuel. As of mid-2018, the supply from Egypt was practically zero.[50] In July 2018, Israel temporarily banned the imports of fuel and gas to pressure Hamas to stop attacks using incendiary kites, further reducing the fuel supply.[51] Thus, despite resumption of power supply from Israel, Gaza's residents have electricity for only four to six hours per day.[52]

---

[46] Joshua Mitnick, "Israel Approves Palestinian Move to Pressure Hamas with Electricity Cuts," *Los Angeles Times*, June 12, 2017.

[47] UNSCO, 2018.

[48] UNSCO, 2018.

[49] Palestine Economic Policy Research Institute, *Palestinian Economic Bulletin*, Bulletin 138, Portland Trust, March 2018.

[50] Office of the Quartet, 2018.

[51] "Israel Cuts Gas, Fuel to Gaza as Egypt Shuts Rafah Gate," 2018.

[52] Hazem Balousha, "Israel Turns the Power Back on to Gaza, Giving Residents About Six Hours' Worth a Day," *Washington Post*, January 7, 2018; Nidal al-Mughrabi, "Palestinian Authority Says Resuming Payment for Gaza's Israeli Electricity," Reuters, January 3, 2018.

Energy Scarcity Impacts on Water and Wastewater Services

The shortage of power and fuel to operate water and wastewater treatment facilities has further reduced Gaza's already limited access to clean water and sanitation solutions. Specifically, it has led to a shortening of the sewage treatment cycle, which means discharging partially treated or untreated sewage into the sea. Lack of power has also put more than 55 wastewater pumping stations in densely populated areas at high risk of flooding, overflow, and contamination and reduced the production rate of 48 small-scale desalination plants to 15 percent of capacity.[53] NGEST, as mentioned, illustrates the extent to which power shortage is an obstacle to water and wastewater services in Gaza. The

Figure 2.5
Lack of Power Makes Wastewater Pumping Stations Vulnerable to Flooding

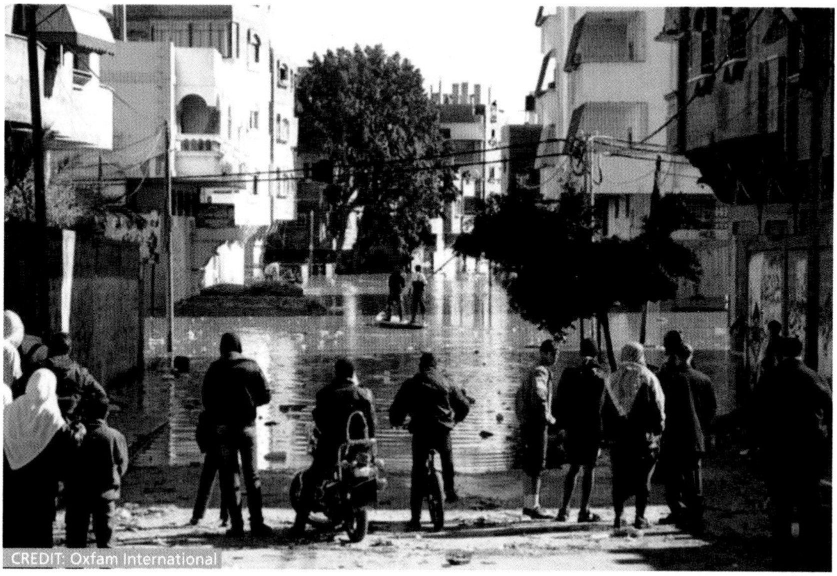

Days after a 2013 thunderstorm, entire neighborhoods in Gaza are still flooded with rainwater and sewage. Efforts to pump water out of the affected areas are prolonged, with people still trapped both inside and outside their houses. Unaltered image licensed through Creative Commons: https://creativecommons.org/licenses/by-sa/4.0/legalcode

---

53 UN, 2017a.

plant became operational in March 2018, but to provide a sustainable long-term wastewater solution to the residents of Northern Gaza, it requires a substantial and dedicated power supply, which is not guaranteed in the long run.[54] Insufficient electricity for wastewater treatment has also led to closure of beaches where raw sewage is dumped directly into the sea.[55]

Another recent impact of the electricity shortage has been on desalination for Gaza's potable water supply. In January 2018, the PWA and GEDCO agreed to provide 1.5 MW per day of electricity needed for the Khan Yunis Short-Term Low-Volume (STLV) desalination plant, which can provide potable water to 75,000 residents of Rafah and Khan Yunis 22 hours per day. However, power shortages as of mid-2018 have limited the plant's operation to only seven hours per day.[56]

In response to the electricity crisis, donors have funded emergency fuel supplies to assist with pressing WASH needs. This funding in 2017 amounted to $4.3 million. However, a sustainable fuel supply is needed in times of emergency, and fuel is not a sustainable solution for Gaza's energy problems. Fuel is expensive and difficult to deliver. Fuel for the GPP is often imported through Egypt, for instance, and thus varies with the security situation in the Sinai and the existence of a safe passage for fuel delivery.[57] To ensure sustainable water, wastewater, and WASH services, power supply in Gaza needs to increase in capacity, diversity of sources, and reliability, which would require substantial investments by all stakeholders to overcome implementation challenges. We discuss specific recommendations to address this problem in Chapter Four.

---

54 Office of the Quartet, 2018.

55 "Municipal Services in Gaza Reduced by 50%," 2018.

56 Office of the Quartet, 2018.

57 UNSCO, 2018.

CHAPTER THREE

Public Health Risks from Water Contamination

Public health experts define the water component of the WASH sector as water quality (important for drinking and cooking); the sanitation component as human excreta disposal; and the hygiene component as comprising both personal hygiene (for cleaning the face, hands, and eyes) and domestic hygiene (for cleaning items in the homes, e.g., food, utensils, floors).[1] The relationship between different WASH components and various diseases has been studied separately and in combination.[2] Inadequate water quality and quantity are associated with different diseases and transmission mechanisms: waterborne transmission of gastrointestinal disease through the fecal-oral route due to poor drinking water *quality* (contaminated water) or inadequate water *quantity* and associated poor hygiene (e.g., contaminated food, fingers, and

---

1 S. A. Esrey, J. B. Potash, L. Roberts, and C. Shiff, "Effects of Improved Water Supply and Sanitation on Ascariasis, Diarrhoea, Dracunculiasis, Hookworm Infection, Schistosomiasis, and Trachoma," *Bulletin of the World Health Organization*, Vol. 69, No. 5, 1991, pp. 609–621.

2 Esrey et al., 1991; L. M. Fry, J. R. Cowden, D. W. Watkins, Jr,, T. Clasen, and J. R. Mihelcic, "Quantifying Health Improvements from Water Quantity Enhancement: An Engineering Perspective Applied to Rainwater Harvesting in West Africa," *Environmental Science and Technology*, Vol. 44, No. 24, 2010, pp. 9535–9541; R. D. Stelmach and T. Clasen, "Household Water Quantity and Health: A Systematic Review," *International Journal of Environmental Research and Public Health*, Vol. 12, No. 6, 2015, pp. 5954–5974.

utensils). Other "water-washed" skin and eye diseases[3] are also associated with inadequate water quantity.[4]

The risk of WASH-associated disease transmission is exacerbated by poor infrastructure and limited access to sufficient improved or clean water sources. Research has shown that young children are particularly vulnerable to WASH-associated disease,[5] compounding the risks in Gaza, where children under age 15 constitute 42.7 percent of the population.[6] Gaza's population density further increases its vulnerability to a disease outbreak.

This section explains how inadequacies in both water quality (stemming from chemical and biological contamination) and water quantity, combined with absence of wastewater treatment, adversely affect public health in Gaza. Moreover, it elaborates on how these inadequacies create additional severe water-related health risks in Gaza and neighboring communities in Israel and Egypt.

It is important to note that the conditions in Gaza are particularly challenging for collecting reliable and current epidemiological data. First, the health care system is fragmented, with four primary providers: the Palestinian Ministry of Health (the Ministry), UNRWA, NGOs, and the private sector. Secondary and tertiary care are provided mainly through the Ministry, while primary care is more fragmented

---

[3] Water-washed diseases are infections that are caused by poor personal hygiene resulting from inadequate water availability. Typical water-washed diseases include Shigella, which causes dysentery, scabies (a highly contagious skin infection), trachoma, yaws, leprosy, conjunctivitis, skin infections and ulcers.

[4] S. Cairncross, "More Water: Better Health," *People and the Planet*, Vol. 6, No. 3, 1997, pp. 10–11.

[5] See, for example, Ciara E. O'Reilly Peter Jaron, Benjamin Ochieng, Amek Nyaguara, Jacqueline E. Tate, Michele B. Parsons, Cheryl A. Bopp, Kara A. Williams, Jan Vinjé, Elizabeth Blanton, Kathleen A. Wannemuehler, John Vulule, Kayla F. Laserson, Robert F. Breiman, Daniel R. Feikin, Marc-Alain Widdowson, and Eric Mintz, "Risk Factors for Death Among Children Less Than 5 Years Old Hospitalized with Diarrhea in Rural Western Kenya, 2005–2007: A Cohort Study," *PLoS Medicine*, Vol. 9, No. 7, 2012, p. e1001256.

[6] Palestinian Central Bureau of Statistics, "Palestine in Figures 2016," Ramallah, Palestine, 2017.

and depends largely on location.[7] The main cities and most villages receive care from the Ministry, while refugees, who make up 1.3 million of Gaza's 2 million residents, receive care from UNRWA. NGOs work in small rural villages, and the private sector provides some primary and secondary care, which is not monitored regularly.[8]

The availability and quality of data from these sources vary, and data are not necessarily standardized. In addition, collecting data in an environment mired in violent conflict is always a challenge, especially where resources are insufficient[9] and electricity is not always available for digital documentation. Reported cases of diarrhea, hepatitis A, and typhoid have been on the rise, but there are many unreported cases of waterborne diseases.[10] It is therefore likely that impacts of the water and wastewater crisis on public health are more severe than current data reflect. Data limitations, however, do not preclude analysis of future risks, which is the focus of this chapter.

Chemical Contamination

Chemical contamination comes primarily from two sources: untreated or undertreated sewage and runoff from fertilizer in agricultural areas. Because the water used by Gaza residents is largely untreated, chemical contaminants such as chloride (Cl-), nitrite (NO_2), and nitrate (NO_3) are often present in drinking water. A 2015 study found that only 12.4 percent of wells in Gaza met WHO standards for nitrate concentration, and only 19.3 percent of wells met WHO standards for chloride

---

7 Khatib et al., 2016.

8 Abdullatif Husseini, Niveen M. E. Abu-Rmeileh, Nahed Mikki, Tarik M. Ramahi, Heidar Abu Ghosh, Nadim Barghuthi, Mohammad Khalili, Espen Bjertness, Gerd Holmboe-Ottesen, and Jak Jervell, "Cardiovascular Diseases, Diabetes Mellitus, and Cancer in the Occupied Palestinian Territory," *The Lancet*, Vol. 373, No. 9668, 2009, pp. 1041–1049.

9 Husseini et al., 2009.

10 United Nations Children's Fund, "Protecting Children from Unsafe Water in Gaza," June 10, 2010.

concentration.[11] Taken together, only 3.6 percent of wells met WHO standards for both chemicals, slightly down from 4 percent the previous year.[12] In addition, an earlier study found that 59 percent of wells in Gaza exceeded the WHO maximum for nitrite concentration.[13] These contaminants present particular risks to children, infants, and pregnant women, who are more susceptible to long-term harm from exposure.[14]

Chloride

Chloride is an anion (negatively charged ion) that makes its way into water sources through both natural and anthropogenic sources, including the use of "inorganic fertilizers, landfill leachates, septic tank effluents, animal feeds, industrial effluents, irrigation drainage, and seawater intrusion in coastal areas."[15] According to WHO standards, the presence of chloride in water sources should be less than 250 milligrams per liter. While healthy adults are generally not considered at risk from a high intake of chloride in drinking water, young children and infants are more susceptible to severe health risks resulting from ingesting high concentrations of chloride.[16] A secondary concern from an elevated presence of chloride in water is its corrosive effects on metal pipes. In large enough concentrations, chloride reacts with the metal

[11] Water Resources Directorate, "2015 Water Resources Status Summary Report/Gaza Strip," Ramallah: Palestinian Water Authority, April 2016.

[12] Water Resources Directorate, 2016.

[13] Medhat Abbas, Maurizio Barbieri, Maria Battistel, Giuditta Brattini, Angelica Garone, and Barbara Parisse, "Water Quality in the Gaza Strip: The Present Scenario," *Journal of Water Resource and Protection*, Vol. 5, No. 1, 2013, pp. 54–63.

[14] Abbas et al., 2013.

[15] WHO, "Chloride in Drinking Water: Background Document for Development," 2003, originally published in *Guidelines for Drinking-Water Quality*, 2nd ed. Vol. 2: *Health Criteria and Other Supporting Information*, Geneva: WHO, 1996.

[16] WHO, 2003 (1996).

ions to create soluble salts, which increase the levels of metals such as lead in drinking water.[17]

If current trends continue, including additional seawater intrusion and reliance on brackish groundwater, the presence of chloride is expected to increase. While the exact health risks of exposure to heavy metals in combination with elevated chloride levels are not completely understood, exposure is thought to be particularly damaging in situations where people or animals are completely dependent on that polluted water source.[18] In Gaza, where a majority of the population depends on contaminated or insufficiently treated groundwater, the health effects could be more severe.

Nitrate and Nitrite

As with chloride, an elevated presence of nitrate and nitrite indicates that the water has been inadequately treated to remove contaminants. Nitrate contamination generally comes from seepage of sewage or nonorganic fertilizer into the groundwater, whereas nitrite can form as the result of chloramination in water distribution systems, rising in concentration as water moves to the extremities of the system. Nitrite can also arise endogenously as the body converts nitrate into nitrite.[19]

In rural or underserved areas, nitrate makes its way into groundwater through nitrogen deposits from fertilizer that is not absorbed by plants. Septic systems, which are often used in areas not connected to a formal sanitary sewer line, can also increase the level of groundwater nitrate because the nitrogen is not completely removed in wastewater and is instead left to percolate into the groundwater.[20] Between 20 and

---

17 WHO Working Group on Sodium, Chlorides, and Conductivity in Drinking-Water, *Sodium, Chlorides, and Conductivity in Drinking-Water: Report on a WHO Working Group, The Hague, 1–5 May 1978*, Copenhagen: WHO Regional Office for Europe, 1979.

18 *Guidelines for Drinking Water Quality*, Third Edition Incorporating the First and Second Addenda, Vol. 1: Recommendations, Geneva: World Health Organization, 2008.

19 WHO, "Nitrate and Nitrite in Drinking-Water," 2016.

20 Margaret McCasland, Nancy M. Trautmann, Keith S. Porter, and Robert J. Wagenet, "Nitrate: Health Effects in Drinking Water," fact sheet, Ithaca, N.Y.: Cornell University Cooperative Extension, 2012.

25 percent of households in Gaza rely on a septic tank or pit system, increasing the risk of elevated nitrate levels to vulnerable populations like infants and people with compromised digestive systems.

Water contamination with nitrate and nitrite poses the most significant health risks to infants under six months old. This happens for several reasons. First, infants have a higher water intake relative to the size of their bodies. Second, infant digestive systems have limited ability to reduce methemoglobin, a non–oxygen-binding form of hemoglobin that causes methemoglobinemia (blue baby syndrome). Finally, infant stomachs' lower acidity promotes the growth of bacteria that convert nitrate to nitrite, which in turn produces methemoglobin.[21] Blue baby syndrome can lead to temporary digestive and respiratory problems or, in extreme instances, brain damage or death.[22] Elevated nitrate levels may also increase the risk of hypertension in children.[23]

A 2008 study conducted by the Helmholtz Center for Environment Research showed that 90 percent of the 115 drinking wells sampled in Gaza contained nitrate in levels two to eight times higher than the maximum for safe drinking water, as determined by WHO.[24] Half of the 640 infants tested in the study showed signs of methemoglobinemia, as well as diarrhea and high blood acidity.[25]

As Figure 3.1 shows, elevated nitrate and chloride levels in Gaza follow slightly different patterns. Nitrate concentrations are highest around population centers, including Gaza City, Deir al Balah, and Rafah. Chloride levels, on the other hand, are elevated in the coastal areas and along the southern portion of the border with Israel. The

---

[21] *Guidelines for Drinking Water Quality, Annex 5: Treatment Methods and Performance*, 4th ed. Geneva: WHO, 2011.

[22] Eran, Bromberg, and Milner, 2014.

[23] Avishalom Pomeranz, Ze'ev Korzets, Daniel Vanunu, Haim Krystal, and Baruch Wolach, "Elevated Salt and Nitrate Levels in Drinking Water Cause an Increase of Blood Pressure in Schoolchildren," *Kidney Blood Pressure Research*, Vol. 23, No. 6, 2000, pp. 400–403.

[24] Basem Shomar, Karsten Osenbrück, and Alfred Yahya, "Elevated Nitrate Levels in the Groundwater of the Gaza Strip: Distribution and Sources," *Science of the Total Environment*, Vol. 398, 2008, pp. 164–174.

[25] Shomar, Osenbrück, and Yahya, 2008.

Figure 3.1
Contour Map of Gaza Coastal Aquifer Nitrate and Chloride Contamination

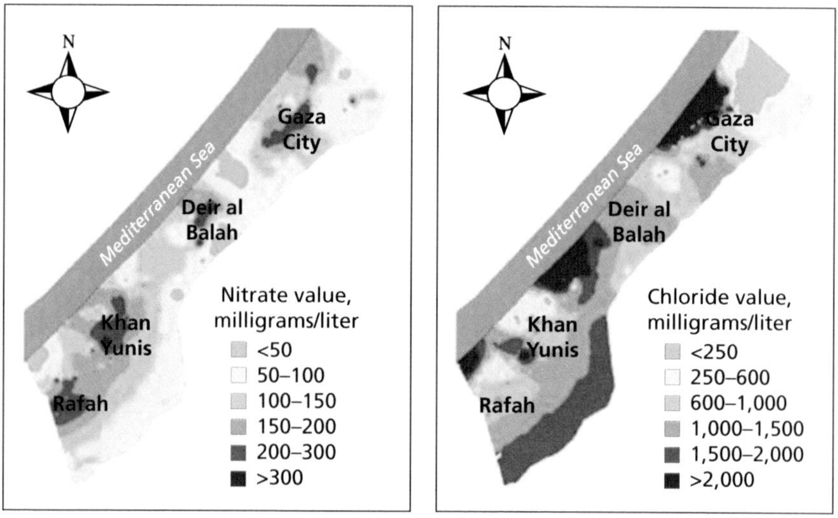

SOURCE: Water Resources Directorate, 2016.

PWA attributes the presence of elevated chloride levels to a reliance on "intensive pumping" from surrounding wells, leading to intrusion of seawater into the water table, while the high nitrate stems from wastewater infiltration.[26]

One solution previously pursued to filter chloride and nitrate out of household water supplies, along with other contaminants, is the distribution and use of point-of-use (POU) reverse osmosis filtering units in Gaza.[27] However, a 2011 UNICEF report found that 20,000 household reverse osmosis units distributed to institutions and facilities that served children were not effectively filtering chemical and microbiological contaminants.[28] To operate at their rated capacity, these units need

---

[26] Water Resources Directorate, 2016.

[27] Reverse osmosis units, even when properly used and maintained, filter out only limited amounts of nitrite, according to the WHO assessment of water treatment methods (WHO, 2016).

[28] *Protecting Children from Unsafe Water in Gaza: Strategy, Action Plan and Project Resources, Summary Documents*, Ramallah, Palestine: UNICEF–Occupied Palestine Territory, 2011.

to be cleaned and disinfected, and some parts need to be replaced regularly. Without access to replacement parts or education on the importance of cleaning and disinfecting the units, the efficacy rate declines significantly. This highlights the need for both better public health education and improved access to filtration systems and other means of removing chemical contaminants from water.

Biological Contamination

Outbreaks of waterborne disease may affect large numbers of people; disease can spread particularly quickly in densely populated areas with inadequate water quantity for personal hygiene and inadequate sanitation infrastructure, especially in people with compromised immune systems. Gaza is one of the most densely populated areas in the world and presents a particular vulnerability to an outbreak of this type.[29] Due to its lack of wastewater treatment and inadequate amounts of water for personal hygiene, the risk of an outbreak of a waterborne or other intestinal disease in Gaza is high.[30]

The most acute risks in Gaza are associated with ingestion of waterborne pathogens via water contaminated with feces from humans or animals. Fecal contamination can be a source of pathogenic bacteria (e.g., cholera, *Salmonella, Shigella*), viruses (e.g., enteroviruses including polio) and parasites (e.g., *Giardia*). Fecal contamination is most likely in areas where wastewater systems are poorly designed or maintained and allow sewage to seep into drinking water from different points in the collection system.[31] Chances of microbiological contamination of water from the aquifer, particularly by fecal coliforms and

29 Michelle Malka Grossman, "Gaza Sewage Crisis is a Ticking Timebomb for Israel," *Jerusalem Post*, March 17, 2016.

30 PWA, "Gaza Strip: No Clean Drinking Water, No Enough Energy, and Threatened Future," March 2014a.

31 Pramod K. Pandey, Philip H. Kass, Michelle L. Soupir, Sagor Biswas, and Vijay P. Singh, "Contamination of Water Resources by Pathogenic Bacteria," *AMB Express*, Vol. 4, No. 1, 2014, p. 51.

fecal *Streptococcus*, increase at each point in the water handling cycle.[32] Private vendors usually supply water through tanker trucks at distribution points in unhygienic conditions. Resulting contaminations lead to significant diarrheal and other water-related disease, not only in Gaza's infants and children under five, but also in the general population.[33]

Insufficient water for personal hygiene (e.g., for handwashing) and contaminated water are already a source of disease in Gaza. In September 2017, the Palestinian Ministry of Health published a report on communicable diseases in Gaza that identified several diseases transmitted through poor personal hygiene and inadequate public infrastructure—among them, acute hepatitis A, typhoid fever, and acute diarrhea.[34] Waterborne diseases and diseases associated with insufficient hygiene are currently a primary cause of illness in children, particularly diarrheal diseases. These diseases have a further indirect effect on a child's ability to absorb nutritional content, leading to higher rates of acute and chronic childhood malnutrition. Poor water quality and access contributed to more than 25 percent of all reported disease in Gaza, and water-related diseases are the primary cause of child morbidity there.[35] Despite a slight decline in the incidence of these diseases, they remain endemic to the area, and some have exhibited an uptick after an initial decline (e.g., typhoid). The data in the report are current as of 2016 and thus do not reflect the epidemiological situation in 2017–2018, during which time infrastructure and living conditions in Gaza deteriorated severely. As mentioned earlier, difficulties in epidemiological data collection[36] could mask more severe public health effects borne out of the water and wastewater crisis.

---

32 Adnan M. Aish, "Drinking Water Quality Assessment of the Middle Governorate in the Gaza Strip, Palestine," *Water Resources and Industry*, Vol. 4, December 2013, pp. 13–20.

33 Eran, Bromberg, and Milner, 2014.

34 "Communicable Diseases in the Gaza Strip—2016," General Directorate of Primary Health Care, Ministry of Health, Palestine, 2016.

35 Ambrogio Manenti, Claude de Ville de Goyet, Corinna Reinicke, John Macdonald, and Julian Donald, *Report of a Field Assessment of Health Conditions in the Occupied Palestinian Territory*, WHO, February 2016.

36 Khatib et al., 2016.

Gaza's young and dense population compounds risks to disease outbreak. The tense geopolitical environment could further complicate the necessary response to such an outbreak.[37]

Bacterial Pathogens

As with chemical contamination, the risk of bacterial contamination in drinking water increases with each additional transfer point before the water reaches the user. For individuals in Gaza who are dependent on water tanks to deliver large quantities of drinking water, this means higher exposure rates to numerous coliform strains, fecal and otherwise, that can cause symptoms including abdominal cramping, bloody diarrhea, vomiting, and fever, among others. Children may risk greater exposure to bacterial contamination through water delivery and storage in schools around Gaza, as a 2016 joint Palestinian Authority and Al Azhar University study found (Figure 3.2).[38] This study was consistent with others that found total and fecal coliform strains present in higher numbers in samples from distribution networks as opposed to samples from wells or home-filtered water.[39]

The prevalence of bacterial contaminants in drinking water is particularly concerning for children, given that UNICEF reported in 2011 that water-associated diseases made up 26 percent of all childhood disease in Gaza and were the leading cause of childhood morbidity.[40] Moreover, the report found that 12 percent of deaths among

---

[37] Eran, Bromberg, and Milner, 2014.

[38] Hossam A. Zaqoot, Mazen Hamada, and Mohammed A. El-Tabash, "Investigation of Drinking Water Quality in the Kindergartens of Gaza Strip Governorates," *Journal of Tethys*, Vol. 4, No. 2, 2016, pp. 88–99.

[39] S. S. Abu Amr and Maged Mohammed Yassin, "Microbial Contamination of the Drinking Water Distribution System and Its Impact on Human Health in Khan Yunis Governorate, Gaza Strip: Seven Years of Monitoring (2000–2006)," *Public Health*, Vol. 122, No. 11, November 2008, pp. 1275–1283.

[40] *Protecting Children from Unsafe Water in Gaza: Strategy, Action Plan and Project Resources, Summary Documents*, 2011.

Figure 3.2
Children May Risk Greater Exposure to Bacterial Contamination Through Water Storage in Schools Around Gaza

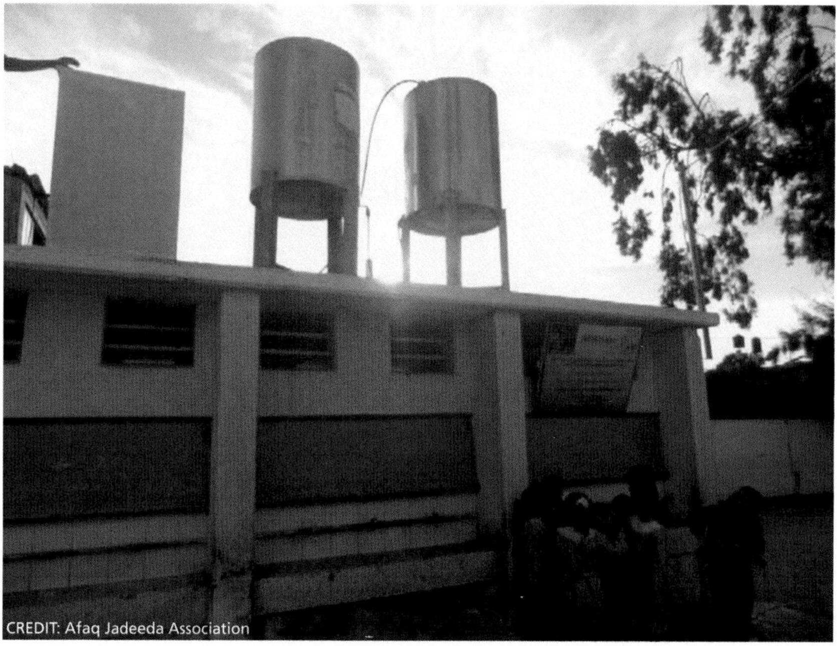

Newly installed water tanks hold large supplies of purified and desalinated water at Bureij Elementary Girls School in Bureij Refugee Camp, Gaza, in 2010. Electricity goes out in Gaza for hours at a time, complicating access to clean water. Unaltered image licensed through Creative Commons: https://creativecommons.org/licenses/by-sa/4.0/legalcode

young children and infants in 2009 were caused by diarrhea, an abundantly treatable and preventable disease.[41]

The risk of a cholera outbreak in particular has been highlighted in recent years.[42] Cholera is acute watery diarrhea caused by ingestion of food or water contaminated with the bacterium *Vibrio cholera*. The massive diarrhea is caused by a toxin produced by the pathogen. Cholera affects both children and adults and can kill within hours to a few

[41] *Protecting Children from Unsafe Water in Gaza: Strategy, Action Plan and Project Resources, Summary Documents*, 2011.

[42] Grossman, 2016.

days if untreated. The mainstay of treatment is rehydration using a specially formulated rehydration solution. Causative factors that contribute to cholera outbreaks are population density, mass gatherings, low access to safe water, and poor sanitation—all conditions that exist in Gaza. Preventive measures, according to the WHO, include the development of piped water systems with water treatment facilities, water filtration, disinfection of water, safe water storage, and construction of systems for safe sewage disposal.[43] All require long-term investment and continued maintenance that are hampered for reasons mentioned earlier.

Viral Pathogens

Transmission of viruses such as enteroviruses in populations with poor personal hygiene and untreated and contaminated water can cause a variety of infections, some of which are mild (such as hand-foot-and-mouth disease) or even asymptomatic. However, some strains of human enterovirus A and B species can have more serious effects, such as viral meningitis. Polio is an enterovirus of great concern, due to the severity of its symptoms, its ability to spread quickly through large populations given the right conditions for transmission, and its status as the target of an ongoing global eradication initiative. Importantly, more than 90 percent of poliovirus infections are asymptomatic, and less than 1 percent result in paralysis; thus, the virus can spread almost silently through large populations. Polio has largely been eradicated in Gaza, as in most of the rest of the world, but viral meningitis—which could have different causes and is apt to spread faster in areas with inadequate water supply and poor personal hygiene—is still one of the most common infectious diseases observed in children in Gaza.[44] Outbreaks are common and have occurred in 1997, 2004, and 2013; infants and children were disproportionately affected each time.[45]

---

[43] WHO, "Cholera," fact sheet, August 2017.

[44] Nedal Ghuneim, Majdi Dheir, and Khaled Abu Ali, "Epidemiology of Different Types of Meningitis Cases in Gaza Governorates, Occupied Palestinian Territory, December 2013–January 2014," *Journal of Antivirals & Antiretrovirals*, Vol. 8, No. 1, 2016, pp. 26–34.

[45] Ghuneim, Dheir, and Abu Ali, 2016.

Rotavirus is another important viral disease affecting Gaza. According to the WHO, rotavirus infection is the most common cause of severe diarrheal disease in children under five years of age.[46] It is spread through fecal-oral contact associated with inadequate personal hygiene. Thus, lack of access to sufficient water for personal hygiene can result in elevated levels of rotavirus infection. A 2006 study found that 28 percent of Gaza children under five years of age who presented with acute gastroenteritis had rotavirus in their stool samples.[47] Rotavirus can be controlled with vaccination; however, the appropriate vaccine was introduced in Gaza only in May 2016.[48] Since then, the number of reported cases of diarrhea in children under three in Gaza has dropped below the five-year average. Even if rotavirus is brought under control with vaccination, however, other causes will ensure that new cases of diarrhea will arise.

Both bacterial and viral pathogens can present a significant health risk not only to people living in Gaza but also to Israeli and Egyptian populations, depending on how the pathogens enter communal water spaces and whether outbreaks are caught early or allowed to spread. Indeed, polio virus has been detected in Israeli sewage systems, attributed to the sewage runoff from Gaza into Israeli waterways—and threatening the success of global eradication efforts.[49]

---

46 World Health Organization, "Rotavirus Vaccines WHO Position Paper—January 2013," *Weekly Epidemiological Record*, Vol. 88, No. 5, 2013, pp. 49–64.

47 F. H. Abu-Elamreen, A. A. Abed, and F. A. Sharif, "Viral, Bacterial and Parasitic Etiology of Pediatric Diarrhea in Gaza, Palestine," *Medical Principles and Practice*, Vol. 17, No. 4, 2008.

48 Majdi Dheir and Nedal Ghuneim, "Communicable Diseases in Gaza Strip: Annual Report," Palestinian General Directorate of Primary Health Care Preventive Medicine, Epidemiology Department, September 2017.

49 Eran, Bromberg, and Milner, 2014, p. 13; it should be noted, however, that both Israel and Egypt have high vaccination rates against polio, making widespread transmission of that disease unlikely. See UNICEF, "Immunization Country Profiles," database, July 2017. UNRWA has shouldered much of the vaccination burden in Gaza, and funding cuts to the agency could lower Gaza's vaccination uptake.

Giardia and Other Intestinal Parasites

As with coliform bacteria, water is more likely to be contaminated with parasites, including protozoa and helminths (worms), as it is transferred from the water distribution center to its eventual destination. Various intestinal parasites (e.g., *Giardia lamblia, Entamoeba histolytica,* and *Cryptosporidium*) cause diarrhea in children, which is in turn associated with higher rates of malnutrition and possible developmental impairments.[50] In one study, 28 percent and 26.7 percent of stool samples from 150 kindergarten children in Gaza were found to have *Entamoeba histolytica* and *Giardia lamblia*, respectively, and 59.2 percent of all examined children were found to suffer from a parasitic infection from one or more parasites.[51]

Rates of intestinal parasites among Gazan children may reach their highest levels in agricultural areas and in neighborhoods with open sewage ponds.[52] A 2011 UNICEF study found that children in Gaza were infected at high rates with both helminths and protozoa, and the younger children most vulnerable to helminths were not receiving deworming treatment typically administered to school-age children in classrooms.[53]

Health Risks Associated with Water Quantity and Hygiene

While much discussion about water and public health centers around water quality, some in the health community have focused on the hygiene and sanitation components of the WASH sector. Water, sanitation, and hygiene are indeed interrelated and often studied together, as

---

[50] Nahed Al Laham, Mansour Elyazji, Rohaifa Al-Haddad, and Fouad Ridwan, "Prevalence of Enteric Pathogen–Associated Community Gastroenteritis Among Kindergarten Children in Gaza," *Journal of Biomedical Research*, Vol. 29, No. 1, January 2015, pp. 61–68.

[51] Al Laham et al., 2015.

[52] Eran, Bromberg, and Milner, 2014, p. 11.

[53] *Protecting Children from Unsafe Water in Gaza: Strategy, Action Plan and Project Resources, Summary Documents*, 2011.

indicated in the discussions earlier related to water contamination and exacerbation of disease spread when water quantity is insufficient for personal and domestic hygiene. This is the case in Gaza, where water supply is estimated at 90 liters per capita per day, below acceptable water quantity standards of 100 liters per capita per day recommended by the WHO.[54]

Some studies have specifically examined water quantity separately from water quality and access (distance to water supplies). Such studies have highlighted the significant role of water quantity on public health. For example, a seminal study from 1991 found a 27-percent median reduction in diarrheal disease morbidity attributable to increased water quantity alone.[55] A modeling study from 2010 looking at the effect of domestic rainwater harvesting in 37 West African cities with a combined population of over 10 million estimated that this quantity-oriented intervention could reduce disability-adjusted life years (a composite index of premature mortality and nonfatal disability) by 9 percent, with POU treatment to improve water quality providing an additional 9-percent reduction.[56]

A more recent systematic review of household water quantity and health indicated different types of improved health outcomes associated with increased water quantity, depending on how the water is used.[57] For example, increased consumption of treated water was associated with reductions in diarrhea and malnutrition associated with *Giardia lamblia* and other diarrheal disease, while increased use for personal hygiene was also associated with reductions in trachoma (a "water-washed" eye disease that can cause blindness). Some health improvements were tied to hygiene interventions such as handwashing education, which underscores the relationship between water (quality), sanitation, and hygiene influencing public health.

---

[54] PWA, GVC Italia, and UNICEF, 2017.

[55] Esrey et al., 1991.

[56] Fry et al., 2010.

[57] Stelmach and Clasen, 2015.

Water, Sanitation, and Hygiene Knowledge, Attitudes, and Practices

A survey that examined the knowledge, attitudes, and practices (KAP) related to WASH was conducted in schools in the Palestinian Territories in 2015.[58] The survey found that in Gaza, the ratio of students to one cleaning staff member (445:1) is more than double that of the West Bank (211:1). These ratios are higher in urban schools. For example, in Khan Yunis, one cleaning staff member serves 553 students. The surroundings of camp-based schools in Gaza were not all hygienic—37 percent of such schools had solid waste and stagnant water. Between 2011 and 2015, there has been a drop in student-to-toilet and student-to–handwashing facility ratios. As Figure 3.3 indicates, on average, there is one toilet for every 71 students in Gaza (versus every 42 students in the West Bank) and one handwashing facility for every 130 students in Gaza (versus every 71 students in the West Bank).[59] The

Figure 3.3
Selected Water Quantity Indicators in Schools, Gaza Versus the West Bank

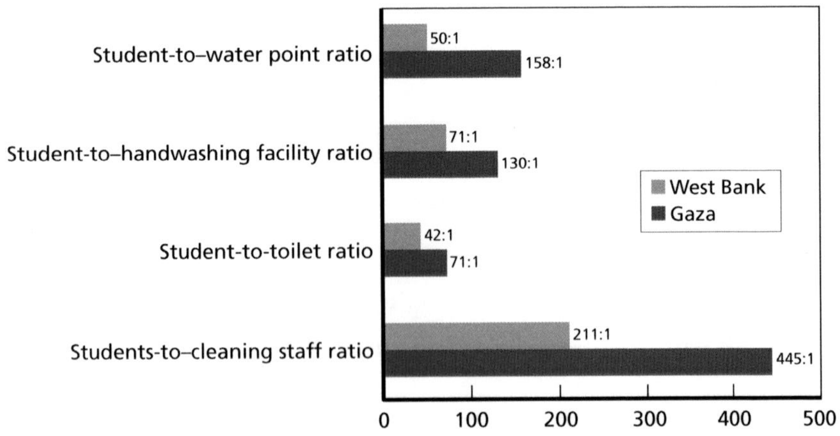

SOURCE: MoEHE, UNICEF in the State of Palestine, and Alpha International, 2016.

58 MoEHE, UNICEF in the State of Palestine, and Alpha International, 2016.

59 MoEHE, UNICEF in the State of Palestine, and Alpha International, 2016.

latter figure is well above the MoEHE guidelines of one handwashing facility for every 30 students.

The student-to–water point (e.g., drinking fountain, faucet) ratio increased in 2015 in Gaza, with one water point for every 158 students (versus every 50 students in the West Bank).[60] The survey was conducted in 2015–2016, before the 2017 deterioration of the water and electricity sectors; thus these figures, which do not meet local and international recommended standards, could be worse as of this writing, raising concerns for schoolchildren's health.

Potential for Waterborne Disease Spread to Israel and Egypt

Gaza's multiple, overlapping water and public health challenges may not stay contained within its boundaries. The combination of poor clean water supply, limited hygiene practices, and insufficient sewage treatment in Gaza could lead to a disease outbreak that spreads outside of Gaza's borders. As noted previously, bacterial and viral pathogens have the potential to travel through sewage and waterways outside of Gaza and thus also present a threat to Israeli and Egyptian populations. The level of risk depends on (1) how the pathogens enter communal water sources; (2) whether a vaccine exists; and (3) if a vaccine is available, whether populations are adequately immunized. The risks increase if vaccination is inadequate or not routinely provided (as with cholera), or if outbreaks are not caught early and are allowed to spread.

Haiti's 2010 cholera epidemic illustrated how easily viral and bacterial pathogens can spread in the right environment. Limited access to clean drinking water left Haitians to drink, wash items in, and bathe in river water contaminated by a strain of cholera from sewage, sickening almost 300,000 people in total and causing over 4,500 deaths in less than five months. Several critical lessons were learned from the Haitian experience, chief among them that the UN and the government of Haiti needed to prioritize long-term investments in piped, treated

---

60 MoEHE, UNICEF in the State of Palestine, and Alpha International, 2016.

drinking water and overall improvements in sanitation throughout the country. The same types of investments are necessary also in Gaza. Additionally, the UN concluded that, in the short to mid term, more emphasis was needed on community and household health programs teaching proper handwashing and hygiene practices, safe disposal of fecal waste, and low-cost water purification techniques.[61] As indicated in the section about WASH KAP, this is an area where intervention could help avert a public health crisis in Gaza.

While health clinics in Gaza might be well-equipped to detect cholera cases early, containment capacity is limited. Although minimal, movement of people and goods between Gaza and Israel, Egypt, and the rest of the world means that if cholera or another epidemic were to spread in Gaza, it might not remain confined there. Cholera outbreaks in Iraq in 2015 and Yemen in 2017 demonstrate that such a scenario is possible in the Middle East.

The risks that Gaza's water problem pose to Israel were first mentioned in Israeli media in 2016 after the Ashkelon desalination plant, which supplies 15 percent to 20 percent of Israel's water, had been shut down periodically due to pollution from Gaza.[62] In May 2017, the Israeli state comptroller issued a report that, for the first time, took on this issue and described water pollution as Israel's most serious cross-border environmental hazard. The comptroller wrote that such widespread pollution not only degrades the groundwater quality of Israel and its neighbors but also harms public health and quality of life. Noting that the government of Israel has yet to formulate a policy for transboundary environmental management with its neighbors, the report called upon the different authorities to join forces to reduce the contamination of resources shared by Israel and the Palestinians, primarily in Gaza.[63]

---

[61] Ana A. Weil, Louise C. Ivers, and Jason B. Harris. "Cholera: Lessons from Haiti and Beyond," *Current Infectious Disease Reports*, Vol. 14, No. 1, 2012, pp. 1–8.

[62] Price, 2016.

[63] State Comptroller, "Zihumei Mayim Bein Medinat Yisrael Le'Shitchey Yehuda, Shomron Ve'Aza [Water Pollutions Between the State of Israel and the Territories of Judea and Samaria and Gaza]," Publication of the Annual Report 67B, 2017, pp. 1481–1583.

The Environmental Protection Ministry welcomed the state comptroller's findings, stressing that "environmental issues do not consider boundaries created by man."[64] In September 2017, Israeli heads of regional councils and leaders of local municipalities in Gaza's vicinity wrote a letter to Prime Minister Benjamin Netanyahu and U.S. Special Envoy for the peace process Jason Greenblatt warning Israel and the United States that Gaza's sewage crisis could lead to the spread of disease. In the letter, which received wide publicity in Israeli press, they wrote:

> Without providing a fundamental and long-term solution to the crisis, it will be coming to our doorstep. In addition to the threats of tunnels, mortars and missiles, we will also be dealing with the pollution of the sea and beaches, pollution of drinking water and pollution of the water of agriculture in the area.[65]

A month later, then–Coordinator of Government Activities in the Territories (COGAT)[66] Major General Yoav (Poli) Mordechai coauthored an article for the INSS describing the dangers the humanitarian situation in Gaza pose for Israeli security and called for a "Marshall Plan" for the strip.[67] In March 2018, Israel's Ministry of Health instructed Israeli farmers in the Gaza vicinity not to use water from two treated-wastewater reservoirs normally used to irrigate their fields, due to contamination by raw sewage from Gaza.[68]

---

64 Sharon Udasin, "Cross-border Water Pollution Threatens Israeli Security, Watchdog Says," *Jerusalem Post*, May 16, 2017.

65 Oren Liebermann and Abeer Salman, "Israeli Mayors Call on US to Solve Gaza's Electricity Crisis," CNN, September 3, 2017.

66 Israeli Defense Ministry unit that coordinates with the international community on all civilian, humanitarian, and infrastructure matters relating to the West Bank and Gaza.

67 Yoav (Poli) Mordechai, Michael Milstein, and Yotam Amitay, "The Next Gaza: The Gaza Strip Between a Dead End and a Glimmer of Hope," *Strategic Assessment*, Vol. 20, No. 3, October 2017.

68 Matan Tzuri, "Gaza Perimeter Agriculture in Peril Due to Water Reservoir Contamination," Ynet News, March 7, 2018.

Medical and Public Health Response Capacity

Gaza's vulnerability to a health crisis does not stem only from the deteriorating WASH infrastructure, insufficient water supply, and the lack of wastewater treatment. Rather, Gaza's overall humanitarian conditions, the Israeli and Egyptian border closure, and the teetering public health sector mean that if an epidemic broke out, containment would be difficult.

The number of doctors, nurses, and hospital beds, relative to the population, declined by 15, 12, and 5 percentage points, respectively, between 2010 and 2017.[69] To cope with the current electricity and water crises, hospitals have reduced cleaning and sterilizing of medical facilities.[70] Gaza's hospitals are operating on generators; any failure could jeopardize the ability of their emergency departments and inpatient units to respond to an epidemic. On January 29, 2018, due to elimination of fuel reserves, the Beit Hanoun hospital, which serves more than 300,000 residents in northern Gaza, announced it would cease delivering medical services.[71]

In September 2018, the UN Humanitarian Fund for the Palestinian territory allocated $1 million to purchase emergency fuel, mainly for backup electricity generators at critical health, water, and sanitation facilities in Gaza "to prevent a complete collapse of services and a potential outbreak of disease." At least an additional $2 million worth of emergency fuel is still needed to maintain minimal health, water, and sanitation services, but donations for emergency fuel were exhausted in early September.[72]

Having not been paid their salaries in months, the 835 cleaning workers at Gaza's hospitals went on strike in February 2018, meaning that garbage has piled up and treatments have stalled.[73] As of Febru-

[69] UN, 2017b.

[70] OCHA, 2017.

[71] UNSCO, 2018.

[72] OCHA, "OPt Humanitarian Fund Releases US $1 Million in Funds to Avoid Collapse of Services in the Gaza Strip; Additional Funds Needed Urgently," September 17, 2018.

[73] "Municipal Services in Gaza Reduced by 50%," 2018.

ary 2018, Gaza's health facilities lacked an estimated 40 percent of essential medicines, including antibiotics, and 32 percent of medical supplies.[74] In addition to funding constraints, lack of coordination and information sharing between the PA, Hamas, and the donor community hinders the effectiveness of health providers in Gaza. According to the UN, the PA health officials do not know in real time the status of medications—whether they are available, missing, or in transit—creating dangerous bottlenecks for addressing medical issues including medication shortages.[75]

In that regard, it is useful to return to cholera as an example outbreak. Addressing a cholera epidemic in real time requires a rapid response and treatment plan, which includes rehydration of patients, access to clean water, and safe food and hygiene practices in households, public places, refugee camps, and hospitals. As of mid-2018, Gaza public health authorities lacked these critical elements for response. In addition, in the event of a cholera outbreak, the complex political situation and the lack of direct communication between all the parties involved could hinder the coordination needed to deliver emergency aid, medicine, and electricity.

The Trump administration's decision to cut funding to UNRWA, the UN fund that supports Palestinian refugees, could further worsen the situation. While critics of UNRWA welcomed this decision and called for folding UNRWA's operations into the United Nations High Commissioner for Refugees (UNHCR), which deals with refugees at large,[76] this proposition is likely not feasible in the short run. First, UNRWA and UNHCR work under distinct mandates, different operational and legal definitions, and separate operational realities, and any change in UNRWA's mandate would require a decision by UN member states. Moreover, UNHCR does not operate in Gaza, where, having been active there for almost 70 years, UNRWA fulfills not only the role of UNHCR but also that of other international organizations,

---

[74] OCHA, 2017.

[75] UNSCO, 2018.

[76] See, for example, Jonathan Greenberg, "Trump's Decision to Cut UNRWA Funding Is the First Step Toward Middle East Peace," *Daily Wire*, January 17, 2018.

such as the WHO and the World Food Programme. It provides critical services and assistance in the areas of food, water, sanitation, hygiene, and health; operates 21 primary health clinics; employs more than 1,000 health staff; and serves more than 4 million annual patient visits.[77] Given the heightened risk of epidemic and the dire status of Gaza's hospitals, UNRWA's clinics and public health network deliver important basic services—including vaccinations to 1.3 million people—and lower the risk of disease outbreaks in Gaza.[78] Reduced capacity at these clinics could heighten the waterborne public health risks in Gaza and surrounding communities in Israel and Egypt.

---

77 UNRWA, 2018.

78 Phone conversation with UN officials based in Jerusalem, March 4, 2018; UNSCO, *Report to the Ad Hoc Liaison Committee*, New York, September 18, 2017.

CHAPTER FOUR

Conclusions and Policy Recommendations

In this chapter, we present the conclusions from our research and introduce policy recommendations for mitigating health risks associated with water insecurity and poor sanitation in Gaza. Given the interconnectedness of the energy, water (drinking, sanitation, and hygiene), and public health sectors, we divide our recommendations into these three broad areas.

Although it is likely that only long-term political solutions will adequately address Gaza's core problems of water and sanitation and consequently mitigate public health risks, there are still near-term actions that could be taken within the existing political environment and constraints to help ease the crisis and reduce the likelihood of a significant public health disaster. In our recommendations, we focus on such near-term steps alongside longer-term suggestions. Several of these recommendations are consistent with initiatives that have already begun or been planned but face implementation challenges. We address implementation issues after introducing the policy recommendations.

Energy Supply Recommendations

The PWA anticipated in 2015 that, by 2017, all water and wastewater projects in Gaza will require 85 MW of power to run effectively.[1] Even if existing desalination, freshwater, and WWTPs were fully oper-

[1] Fanack Water of the Middle East and North Africa, "Increasing Water Availability in Gaza," June 5, 2015.

ational, inconsistent supplies of fuel and electricity limit their capacity, and lack of consistent supply hinders the completion of new water and wastewater projects.[2] As a result, the first step in addressing Gaza's urgent water and sanitation deficits is to increase the quantity and consistency of Gaza's electricity supply. Specific steps to help achieve this goal are detailed next. Beyond political complexities, the key challenge with most ideas, except for ensuring consistent fuel supply, is that they require long-term investments that, even if implemented today, will be viable only in the long run and thus unable to address Gaza's current challenges.

Ensure Consistent and Reliable Supply of Fuel for Critical Facilities

As explained earlier, the PA-imposed tax on fuel imports amounts to 100 percent of refined fuel prices. Consequently, due to the Fatah-Hamas dispute over the taxation issue, fuel imports for the GPP enter Gaza via the Rafah crossing from Egypt (fuel delivered by UNRWA and other international organizations to power their facilities, as well as fuel imports by private vendors, enter Gaza through the Kerem Shalom crossing from Israel).[3] Hence, fuel imports for the GCC do not only hinge on the ability to fund fuel purchases (which is discussed next as part of the public health solutions) but also on ensuring that a safe passage is available for transferring fuel into Gaza from Egypt. In addition, the PA should consider tax exemptions on fuel purchased from Israel so that the GPP fuel supply does not depend solely on imports from Egypt.

Fuel reserves at the GPP, which can hold some two days' worth of fuel, sufficient to produce 25 MW per day (350,000 liters), should

2 Roundtable with subject-matter experts, Tel Aviv, May 25, 2017; one of the repeating themes in conversations with subject-matter experts is that although donors might be willing to fund the construction of projects, they are unwilling to commit to footing energy bills in perpetuity and thus hold back until consistent energy supply is guaranteed before beginning or completing projects.

3 Gaza expert, email exchange with authors, June 14, 2018.

be expanded to enable fuel storage for at least several days when fuel imports are disrupted.[4]

As noted, emergency fuel supplies for generators powering critical health, water, and sanitation facilities in Gaza are dwindling quickly. Donors should ensure continued support for emergency fuel supplies to maintain basic services (according to the United Nations, 950,000 liters of emergency fuel are needed every month to sustain life-saving services in Gaza).[5]

Invest in Solar Projects

One of the initiatives advanced by the international community is a $12 million rooftop solar power array for the Gaza Industrial Estate, a large business area. If executed and implemented as planned, the project will be completed in 2019 and will provide power to the 32 businesses in the industrial area at a lower price than fuel-based generation.[6] In June 2018, the U.S. administration was reportedly seeking funding from Arab Gulf countries to advance the construction of a solar energy project near the Egyptian town of El-Arish in northern Sinai that would serve some of Gaza's energy needs.[7] However, Egypt conditioned its agreement on the PA resuming authority in Gaza. Instead, Israel has approved a similar plan to build a solar field on Israeli territory by the Erez Crossing, which will be funded by "private Israeli and foreign elements." Citing security concerns, Israeli authorities have said this field will not provide employment for workers from Gaza.[8]

Solar projects have the potential to address Gaza's power dependence on high-cost fuel imports, and thus the international community and business sector should consider investment in utility-scale solar

---

4 UNSCO, 2018b.

5 OCHA, 2018.

6 "Solar Power Brightens Gaza's Business Prospects," Environment News Service, March 15, 2018.

7 Amir Tibon and Amos Harel, "Trump Administration Will Ask Gulf States to Invest up to $1 Billion in Gaza Economy," *Haaretz*, June 17, 2018.

8 Alex Fishman, "Israel Approves Solar Field to Increase Power Supply to Gaza," Ynet News, June 27, 2018.

power. Another advantage of solar power is that it requires a single large investment but not regular payment collection, which could help overcome the governance vacuum hindering progress on other electricity solutions.[9]

Solar power could also help make lifeline infrastructure more resilient. For example, primary health clinics providing relatively simple services could be powered by solar energy,[10] allowing the reservation of limited available electricity for critical facilities. The UN estimates the cost of operating the 56 Ministry of Health–run primary health clinics with solar power at $8.9 million.[11] Coordination between stakeholders and donors could advance this approach and help sustain medical services in Gaza. Other solar projects, for example, include an EU-funded photovoltaic solar field designed to provide 0.5 MW of electricity per day to fuel the Southern Gaza Desalination Plant, which could provide drinking water for up to 250,000 people in Southern Gaza by 2020.[12]

An additional solar initiative is MIT's solar-powered brackish water desalination plants for the production of potable water.[13]

Upgrade Electricity Transmission and Distribution Network

In parallel to other proposed solutions, the electricity transmission and distribution network in Gaza is in urgent need of maintenance and repair. In the long run, it needs to be expanded and upgraded to enable additional and diverse domestic generation capacity and imports to be brought online in Gaza.

---

[9] Discussion with former UN official working in Gaza, Washington, D.C., June 4, 2018.

[10] Daniel K. Eisenbud, "World Bank to Help Fund Solar Panels Project in Gaza," *Jerusalem Post*, August 1, 2017.

[11] UNSCO, 2018b.

[12] Office of the European Union Representative, "Water for Gaza: EU Switches on the Biggest Solar Energy Field in the Gaza Strip to Fuel Projects Providing Drinking Water to People in Dire Need," August 2, 2018.

[13] Devarajan Ramanujan, Natasha Wright, Sebastian Truffaut, Gregor von Medeazza, and Amos Winter, "Sustainability Analysis of PV-Powered Electrodialysis Desalination for Safe Drinking Water in the Gaza Strip," in *IDA 2017 World Congress on Water Reuse and Desalination*, 2017.

While not the main source of power supply, the three power lines from Egypt, which could provide Gaza with 20 to 30 MW of electricity per day, need to be upgraded as well. Recall that the failure of these lines in the summer of 2017 exacerbated the overall energy crisis.[14] The lines were partially repaired since then but as of August 2018 continue to be unreliable and provide virtually no electricity.[15] An additional 25 MW per day could be available from Egypt by mid-2019, according to the Quartet.[16] Replacing existing feeder lines could upgrade the connection with Egypt, and electricity imports could be doubled to almost 50 MW per day.[17]

Advance the "161kV Line"

Israel, the PA, and the international community should continue advancing the construction of the "161kV Line" that will establish a high-voltage connection between Gaza and the Israel Electric Corporation grid. This would allow approximately an additional 100 MW per day of electricity to flow into Gaza within a few years. The additional electricity supply would support the operation of Gaza's water and/or WWTPs. The cost of constructing the 161kV Line is estimated by the Palestinian Energy and Natural Resources Authority at $45 million,[18] though PWA would incur additional costs to purchase the electricity and operate the plants more regularly.

Despite international pledges to support Gaza's stabilization, donors have thus far not offered to fund the 161kV Line. Like other investments in the energy sector in Gaza, investment in the 161kV Line depends on guarantees of sufficient supply and enforcement of payment, control, and appropriate management of the network. These

---

14 Gisha—Legal Center for Freedom of Movement, "Egyptian Power Supply Lines to Gaza to Resume Operations After Being Shut Down for Two Months," September 7, 2017.

15 "Gaza's Only Power Plant Stops Work Due to Lack of Fuel," *Middle East Monitor*, April 13, 2018.

16 Office of the Quartet, 2018.

17 UNSCO, 2018b.

18 Office of the Quartet, "Energy," fact sheet, undated.

remain challenging as long as the PA and Hamas are in dispute.[19] In addition, substantial parts of the works for the 161kV Line are required on Israel's side of the border, and the international community is reluctant to fund projects in Israel (as in other advanced economies).[20] Nevertheless, the international community should work with Israel and the PA to design a feasible implementation plan to help ensure construction of this important line in the long run.

Connect Gaza to Natural Gas Infrastructure

The 161kV Line could be an important medium-term step to help meet Gaza's energy needs. In the long run, a potential solution to Gaza's energy woes would be to connect it to natural gas infrastructure for the purpose of supplying new gas-fired power plants. The option proposed currently is construction of a gas pipeline connecting the GPP to the Israeli natural gas network, which would allow the plant to operate at 140 MW per day (up from 0 to 25 MW as of mid-2018).[21] Technically speaking, by mid-2021 gas-based power generation for Gaza could increase to some 600 MW per day. Domestic power generation is essential for major water projects, including the Central Desalination Program currently in planning stages.[22]

Ensure Independent and Sufficient Power Supply to New Wastewater Treatment and Desalination Plants

Overcoming electricity shortages is vital not only for future projects in the water, wastewater, and WASH sectors but also to enable sustained operation of existing infrastructure that would bring substantial improvement in basic service provision for Gaza's residents. NGEST, for example, became operational in March 2018, but its sustainable operation requires consistent energy supply, which may not be secure.[23]

---

[19] Office of the Quartet, undated.

[20] Conversation with UN officials, Jerusalem, July 13, 2018.

[21] Conversation with UN officials, Jerusalem, July 13, 2018.

[22] Office of the Quartet, 2018.

[23] "North Gaza Communities Will Finally Benefit from Sewage Treatment Services," World Bank, March 12, 2018.

In parallel, GEDCO and the PWA signed a memorandum of understanding (MoU) to ensure that the required energy from the existing electricity network is delivered to the plant. This MoU, however, has not been implemented as of summer 2018. It is critical to ensure the MoU is implemented and see whether the dedicated line established for NGEST provides sufficient electricity to the plant to enable its efficient operation independent from other energy sector improvements.

In terms of potable water supply, a similar dedicated power supply should be considered to enable the operation Khan Yunis STLV desalination plant, with 1.5 MW required for the plant to operate 22 hours per day.[24]

Water Sector Recommendations

We divide our policy recommendations for the water sector into several areas: increasing potable water supply through additional water purchases, desalination, or other treatment options at the industrial or household level; improving the water transmission and distribution network; and investing in wastewater solutions. Many of these solutions depend in large part on sufficient electricity supply, as described previously.

Increase Safe Water Supply

Increase Amount of Purchased Water

As mentioned earlier, in July 2017, the PA and Israel reached an understanding on water whereby the PA would be able to buy an additional 33 mcm of potable water per year from Israel, of which 10 mcm would be delivered to Gaza. Based on the capacity of the existing pipelines, Israel could provide the first 5 mcm of water immediately. Further investments, however, are needed to build a new pipeline connecting Israel to Gaza to supply the remaining 5 mcm. While the two sides have agreed on the price and quantity, as of summer 2018, there has

[24] "North Gaza Communities Will Finally Benefit from Sewage Treatment Services," 2018.

not been a formal agreement.[25] It is important that both sides take the necessary measures to ensure that the allocated water is quickly supplied to Gaza, including facilitation and prioritization of any infrastructure upgrades that may be needed. For that, Israel and the PA need to finalize the agreement and reassert their commitment to this project, and Israel will need to quickly authorize the materials required, even if some are on the dual-use list.

Once the agreement is fully implemented, Gaza would purchase a total of 20 mcm per year. The imported water could be blended with groundwater, making 40 mcm of potable water available.[26] Though we acknowledge that this amount would still not meet demand in Gaza, it would still represent an increase over previous agreements.

Improve the Water Storage and Distribution System

One of the limiting factors of the amount of water that can be sold to Gaza from Israel is infrastructure: the lack of storage capacity and the poor conditions of the existing transmission and distribution pipe system. Additional storage capacity and urgent investment to reduce network losses are necessary. Following the completed refurbishment of the al-Muntar reservoir in Gaza City by KFW,[27] donors could be further encouraged to build an additional reservoir to accommodate water imported from Israel. In addition, repairs to the distribution system or additional household connections could help to ensure that treated water reaches residents. For example, the PWA has completed the design of the associated works for the Gaza desalination project, which will improve the transportation and distribution of additional water from Israel, the small desalination plants, and the central Gaza desalination plant. The cost of this project is $220 million, $60 million of which is available from Kuwait.[28]

---

[25] PWA official, 2018.

[26] EcoPeace Middle East, "Brief—Gaza's Water and Sanitation Crisis and Implications for Regional Stability," February 2016.

[27] EcoPeace Middle East, 2016.

[28] PWA official, 2018.

Facilitate and Advance the Development of Desalination Plants

In January 2017, a new desalination plant opened in Deir el-Balah in central Gaza. Assuming a consistent energy supply, in its initial stage the plant is supposed to produce 6,000 cubic meters of water per day (2.2 mcm per year), satisfying a small fraction of Gaza's total water demand.[29] The international community should continue investing in the second stage that is meant to double capacity by 2019, again assuming available electricity to power the plant.

Furthermore, in January 2018, the PWA announced plans to build a central desalination plant in Khan Yunis in southern Gaza.[30] In March 2018, donors pledged 456 million euros for the plant and its associated works but have not yet followed through on these commitments.[31] This plan, like other infrastructure projects, faces implementation challenges discussed later in this chapter. Specific additional challenges include the need to also build distribution lines and pumping stations, along with broader repairs to the distribution network to ensure that water from the desalination plant reaches residents.[32] Nonetheless, given that desalination is one of the only ways to guarantee Gaza's water needs are met in the long term, these plans should be advanced and implementation challenges fully addressed. In addition, research and development should be conducted to develop solar-powered desalination plants that could guarantee consistent water supply even if the energy crisis is not fully solved.

Invest in Other New Treatment at the Industrial or Household Level

In addition to desalination, there are water treatment solutions that can help mitigate the waterborne hazards in Gaza. Table 4.1 summarizes various treatment approaches and indicates whether a mitigation option listed in a given row is applicable for controlling the hazard

---

29 Fares Akram, "Desalination Plant Opens to Bring Gaza Some Relief," *Times of Israel*, January 19, 2017.

30 "Palestinian Water Authority Announces Plans for Desalination Plant in Gaza," Ma'an News Agency, January 31, 2018.

31 PWA official, 2018.

32 European Commission, undated.

Table 4.1
Water Treatment Options for Waterborne Health Hazards in Gaza

Treatment	Use Setting	Chloride	Nitrate	Nitrite	Bacteria	Viruses	Protozoa	Description
Bank filtration	Industrial			■	■	■	■	Low-cost way of cleaning surface water by removing both particulates and microorganisms. Done by passing surface water through alluvial sediments (by drilling boreholes adjacent to the source).
Biological denitrification	Industrial		■					Uses naturally occurring bacteria to consume nitrate in groundwater and convert it to nitrogen gas. Removes nitrate from wastewater. Use in drinking water possible but rare.
Chlorination	Industrial and household			■	■	■	■	Adding chlorine gas or one of several chemical compounds to water. Chlorine is used primarily as a disinfectant but also acts as an oxidant that can decompose or oxidize dissolved contaminants to more easily removable forms.
Ion exchange	Industrial and household		■	■				Ions of same charge exchanged between water containing dissolved contaminants and a substance called ion exchange resin, substituting a less-objectionable substance for the contaminant. Used in water-softening.

Table 4.1—Continued

Treatment	Use Setting	Chloride	Nitrate	Nitrite	Bacteria	Viruses	Protozoa	Description
Ozonation	Industrial and household							Ozone, a powerful oxidant, used as a primary disinfectant. Also reacts with natural organics to increase their biodegradability and is thus effective for the degradation of a wide range of pesticides and other organic chemicals.
Reverse osmosis/ membrane filtration	Industrial and household							Processes based on separation of contaminant particles from water by means of membranes. Distinction made between nanofiltration and low-pressure processes (ultrafiltration, microfiltration), which is often a step before or used in conjunction with high-pressure reverse osmosis, used for desalination of brackish water.
UV irradiation	Industrial and household							Uses ultraviolet light, alters the DNA of microorganisms in water and halts their reproduction and inactivates them. Effective against bacteria, viruses, protozoans.

Table 4.1—Continued

Treatment	Use Setting	Chloride	Nitrate	Nitrite	Bacteria	Viruses	Protozoa	Description
Ceramic filtration	Household				■		■	A flowerpot-shaped ceramic filter impregnated with colloidal silver is filled with water, which seeps through to a treated-water receptacle. Ceramic filters are used primarily for the removal of protozoa and bacterial pathogens.[a]
Slow sand filtration	Household			■	■		■	Water passed through a tank up to 1.5m deep containing sand. Turbidity and microorganisms are separated in the top 5cm of the sand layer, while treated water flows through to be collected in underdrains at the bottom of the filter.[b]

NOTES: Shaded cell indicates a given method is effective for that contaminant type.

[a] U.S. Centers for Disease Control and Prevention, "Ceramic Filtration," March 21, 2012a.

[b] U.S. Centers for Disease Control and Prevention, "Slow Sand Filtration," fact sheet, March 21, 2012b.

listed in a given column (shaded cells), or ineffective against the risk in that column (white cells). For example, biological denitrification is effective at reducing the levels of nitrate in the water; however, it does not reduce the presence of chloride. The mitigation methods listed can be suitable either for industrial use (e.g., in water treatment plants) or for household deployment. The second column in the table specifies the typical use setting for a given method. Some methods, like reverse osmosis, can be used in multiple settings. A brief description of each mitigation method is provided in the table.[33]

As the number and distribution of shaded cells indicate, many of these methods can help address health risks from Gaza's polluted water, but no single method is sufficient for all. Therefore, these methods should be considered in combination. Reverse osmosis or membrane filtration can be highly effective in removing chemical contamination but is also the most expensive and energy-intensive approach. Given Gaza's intermittent energy supply, less energy-dependent options are preferable. Conversely, the least expensive and most centralized option to address biological contamination and nitrate would be chlorination, yet, implemented in isolation, that does not address nitrate or chloride contamination.

Ceramic and sand filtration can be implemented fairly easily at the household level, but such a solution could not be effectively monitored by a central water or public health institution (although one could provide the necessary training and education). These filtration methods do not, however, address nitrate, chloride, and viruses, which account for some of Gaza's most severe health hazards. Thus, if adopted at the household level, these approaches would need to be accompanied by water boiling and/or household chlorination, the latter of which could then risk overchlorination when unsupervised. Likewise, chlorination and ion exchange can be effective for some issues at the household level but would need to be paired with education and training on how to clean systems and change filters.

---

[33] Except where noted otherwise, based on *Guidelines for Drinking Water Quality*, 2011, Annex 5: Treatment Methods and Performance.

This brief comparison shows that at least some additional treatment approaches could be viable for addressing some of Gaza's waterborne health risks. However, the trade-offs presented here should be examined more thoroughly. More research is needed to assess the feasibility of adopting these methods in the context of Gaza and prioritize them based on benefits, cost, dependence on equipment and materials that are considered dual-use, and other implementation considerations.

Distribute Chemicals and Spare Parts for Existing Household Treatment Systems

Other interim solutions to ensure that Gaza's residents drink clean water include providing chemicals for water treatment and disinfection, spare parts for existing POU filters, and hygiene kits that could be distributed to vulnerable households in Gaza. Even though these materials may be on Israel's dual-use list, this may be a necessary approach to prevent outbreaks of waterborne disease in advance of a long-term solution. They could be provided either by the Palestinian government (e.g., PWA, Health Ministry) or by the donor community.

Wastewater Treatment Solutions

As noted earlier, Gaza's most urgent near-term need in terms of wastewater treatment is a reliable and sufficient electricity supply to run existing WWTPs and pumps for the approximately two-thirds of Gaza's population with sewer connections. If the electricity supply is resolved, additional near- to long-term recommendations could help resolve the sanitation concerns while simultaneously addressing groundwater depletion.

Construct Additional WWTPs

As of summer 2018, at least three new WWTPs are under construction or near completion in Gaza, including the completed NGEST in northern Gaza. The plant, which has a capacity of 35,600 cubic meters per day, is designed to serve the northern area of Gaza, where some 33,000 cubic meters of wastewater are generated per day. Another is the Khan Yunis WWTP, which is under construction and has a capacity of 26,000 cubic meters per day. As of March 2018, the PWA has been trying to raise funds for this plant; if funding is available, construction could be completed by mid-2019. The third plant is the Central Gaza WWTP, located east of Al Bureij and Wadi Gaza, which is under construction with funding from KFW. The plant capacity is 60,000 cubic meters per day, and it is expected to be completed in mid-2019 as well.[34]

First and foremost, these plants are intended to treat sewage already flowing into the wastewater system from existing connections, particularly in densely populated areas. Completing these major projects is an urgent near-term priority. Fully operational, NGEST, Khan Yunis WWTP, and the Central Gaza WWTP could provide an additional 94,600 cubic meters per day of wastewater treatment, substantially reducing the flow of untreated sewage.

Use Treated Wastewater to Recharge Coastal Aquifer

A complementary solution to new wastewater treatment is to use treated effluent to recharge groundwater in the coastal aquifer. Treated wastewater of sufficiently high quality could help to offset unsustainable withdrawals, prevent further seawater intrusion, and potentially reduce chloride and nitrogen levels in the aquifer. This concept is already incorporated into NGEST, where the treated effluent will be infiltrated in the same infiltration basins that used to receive partially treated effluent from the old WWTP in Beit Lahia but now can receive cleaner effluent from the new plant. In parallel, as of March 2018, construction of 15 recovery wells, a storage tank, and a pumping station was ongoing to enable recovery and reuse of the treated effluent.[35] Such systems could be further expanded to newly built or existing WWTPs, providing co-benefits for both sustainable clean water supply and wastewater sanitation.

Repair the Wastewater Collection System and Connect Additional Residents

The sewage collection network currently services only two thirds of Gaza's population and is in a state of disrepair. As with electricity and

---

[34] PWA official, 2018.

[35] PWA official, 2018.

water supply, repairs to the collection and conveyance sanitary sewer system are needed and could reduce the flow of untreated sewage into surface waters or groundwater. Furthermore, a long-term recommendation would be to connect additional residential customers to the wastewater system, reducing the use of potentially unsafe cesspits and open drains.

Public Health Recommendations

The public health and health care sectors in Gaza are near collapse for a variety of reasons, including but not limited to insufficient donor funding, restrictions on access to and movement of medical supplies and medicines, an economic crisis, and a governance vacuum hindering coordination between health authorities and providers in Gaza and the West Bank. Here, we focus on public health recommendations that could mitigate waterborne health challenges. Specifically, we divide our recommendations into the need to prevent or respond to a disease outbreak, including planning for such an outbreak and ensuring that proper epidemiological mitigation capacity exists in such a scenario; maintaining basic health services in Gaza, including international funding for clinics and physicians, and sustaining energy supply to hospitals; and promoting rigorous hygiene and sanitation education.

Prevent or Respond to a Disease Outbreak

In addition to the options recommended in Table 4.1 to mitigate waterborne health hazards and the broader interventions to improve water quality and quantity described earlier, we recommend that specific attention be given to the risk of a cholera outbreak occurring in Gaza as an illustration of the type of public health response that would be needed.

Efforts should not only focus on broad preventive measures such as clean water, sanitation, and hygiene practices, but health authorities and the donor community should also preemptively distribute cholera vaccinations and WHO/UNICEF rehydration salt packets in Gaza through clinics and hospitals, which have successfully secured vaccination uptake of near 100 percent.[36] Note that cholera vaccine provides only partial and temporary protection, and it takes time to work once an individual is vaccinated. This means that, at best, vaccination can limit further disease transmission after several weeks if enough people are vaccinated.[37]

Ensure Adequate Capacity to Promptly Respond to and Contain a Waterborne Disease Outbreak

Local and international health authorities must also ensure adequate epidemiological and medical capacity to promptly respond to and contain a cholera or other waterborne or water-related disease outbreak. Despite the political challenges, there may be a foundation for partnership that could, with appropriate political will, be harnessed. For example, the longstanding partnership among the State of Palestine, Israel, and Jordan through the Middle East Consortium on Infectious Disease Surveillance (MECIDS) is a self-organized partnership that has tackled infectious disease issues of common interest to its members, ranging from laboratory diagnosis of selected foodborne pathogens to pandemic influenza preparedness.[38] Gaza has not participated in this partnership, but, despite the political challenges, all relevant stakeholders should take advantage of existing partnerships such as MECIDS.

Plan for an Outbreak Scenario

According to an Egyptian security official, on the Egyptian side at present there is no preparation for a disease outbreak scenario.[39] Comprehensive preparation for such a disaster is lacking at other levels as well—between different stakeholders and among the donor commu-

---

[36] WHO, *Gaza Strip: Joint Health Sector Assessment Report*, Health Cluster in the occupied Palestinian territory, Gaza, September 2014. Because UNRWA provides vaccinations to Palestinian refugees, it is important to examine whether funding cuts could undermine vaccination uptake in Gaza.

[37] Melinda Moore, "Cholera in Haiti: No Surprise This Time Around," *Inside Sources*, October 27, 2016.

[38] Middle East Consortium on Infectious Disease Surveillance, "Welcome Message," homepage, undated.

[39] Discussion with senior Egyptian security official, Tel Aviv, Israel, March 14, 2018.

nity, for instance.[40] Given the magnitude of this threat, the international community, Israel, Egypt, the PA, and relevant stakeholders should form a special task force that would prepare an action plan to implement immediate and mid-term responses to prevent a disease outbreak and to contain it if such an outbreak occurs. One useful way to prepare for such a scenario is through simulations and tabletop exercises that can identify and address important gaps in the ability of local and international stakeholders to respond to a public health emergency in a coordinated way.[41]

Maintain Basic Health Services

A second set of public health recommendations focuses on maintaining basic health services in Gaza, by both sustaining UNRWA's operations in Gaza and continuing the donor supply of fuel to hospitals and clinics.

Sustain UNRWA's Public Health Operations in Gaza

The United States should consider revisiting its funding cuts to the Palestinians and to UNRWA. In the meantime, the donor community should step in and bridge funding gaps to ensure that the U.S. cuts do not further undermine UNRWA's public health operations in Gaza, which provide vaccination and other public health and medical services. Israeli officials were reportedly aware of this issue and had asked the United States not to cut humanitarian funding in the West Bank and Gaza.[42]

Continue Supplying Fuel to Hospitals

While longer-term solutions are designed, donors should continue supplying fuel to hospitals and critical infrastructure to avoid a total collapse of services. After UN Security Council Special Coordinator for

---

[40] Discussion with WHO official based in Gaza, Washington, D.C., June 4, 2018.

[41] As a concrete example, MECIDS has already approached pandemic influenza preparedness this way.

[42] Barak Ravid, "Netanyahu Wants to Transfer Part of UNRWA Funding to Jordan," Axios, March 8, 2018; conversation with Israel Defense Forces official, Tel Aviv, July 12, 2018.

the Middle East Peace Process Nickolay Mladenov warned in late January 2018 that funding for continued fuel supply would not be sufficient beyond February,[43] Qatar and the United Arab Emirates (UAE) pledged $11 million (Qatar $9 million and the UAE $2 million) for emergency hospital generators.[44] But these interventions, too, lasted for only a few months, and continued funding is needed until regular electricity supply is restored.

Improve WASH Infrastructure, Practices, and Education in Schools

A third public health recommendation for Palestinian health authorities and the international donor community is to invest in improving WASH facilities, practices, and education in schools. The need to improve WASH education was identified in the 2011 KAP survey described in Chapter Three.[45] Since then, several interventions have sought to provide a growing number of students access to safe drinking water, sanitation facilities, and education for good hygiene. The follow-on survey conducted in 2015 showed improvement in the availability of WASH infrastructure in schools; hygiene education activities; and the participation of teachers, parents, and students in such activities, as well as changes in KAP of students related to hygiene behavior.[46] However, the survey results clearly demonstrate that more needs to be done.

Invest in WASH Infrastructure in Schools

First, as noted in Chapter Three, WASH infrastructure in Gazan schools is severely inadequate, with a lack of access to toilets, handwashing facilities, and drinking-water points. The 2015 KAP survey also found lack of cleanliness, soap, toilet paper, sanitary pads, and door locks in bathrooms.[47] In Gaza's schools, the student-to-toilet, student-to–hand-

---

43 UNSCO, "Nickolay Mladenov Special Coordinator for the Middle East Peace Process: Briefing to the Security Council on the Situation in the Middle East," January 25, 2018a.

44 Nidal al-Mughrabi, "UAE, Qatar Donate Funds to Stave off Gaza Health Crisis," Reuters, February 9, 2018c.

45 MoEHE, UNICEF in the State of Palestine, and Alpha International, 2016.

46 MoEHE, UNICEF in the State of Palestine, and Alpha International, 2016.

47 MoEHE, UNICEF in the State of Palestine, and Alpha International, 2016.

washing facility, and student-to–water point ratios are all well above Palestinian government and international standards.[48] Thus, continued improvement of WASH infrastructure in schools, where vulnerable young populations are concentrated, is of prime importance. The Palestinian government and the international community should continue investing in WASH facilities in schools; supervise the status and cleanliness of these facilities, perhaps through frequent and regularly scheduled visits; and ensure that school administrations are equipped and trained in how to maintain cleanliness and provide supplies such as toilet paper and soap.

Promote WASH Training and Education

Another recommendation that emerges from analyzing the results of the KAP surveys conducted in 2011 and 2015 is the need for hygiene education and training. While fewer teachers reported needing training to promote good WASH practices in 2015 compared with 2011, 40 percent of the teachers still reported a need for such training. Similarly, while many more students were aware of hygiene practices in 2015 than in 2011, the responses indicate an alarming lack of knowledge about what constitutes good hygiene.[49] It is therefore important that Palestinian health authorities sustain and strengthen hygiene education in schools and, ideally, extend this education to the students' personal networks, whose members may not have developed the proper WASH KAP. This is especially important in schools located within refugee camps or areas without proper WASH infrastructure. Teacher training on hygiene education should be enhanced to facilitate expansion of such education programs. These steps are feasible even under current conditions and resource constraints.

---

[48] MoEHE, UNICEF in the State of Palestine, and Alpha International, 2016.

[49] MoEHE, UNICEF in the State of Palestine, and Alpha International, 2016.

Addressing Implementation Challenges

The water-energy-health crisis in Gaza represents a failure of governance. Its key underlying problems could be fully addressed in the long term through greater investment in water and wastewater treatment infrastructure and new power infrastructure, along with greater water or electricity purchases from outside Gaza. These are all achievable with existing technologies. Instead, the current barriers to policy solutions are largely political. The complex political dynamic in the region between Israel and Hamas, the intra-Palestinian rivalry between Hamas and the PA, and tension with Egypt all represent barriers to overcome. Reconciliation between the Fatah-dominated PA and Hamas was thought of as means to alleviate some of the WASH and energy challenges, but as of August 2018, reconciliation was stalled and the process had yet to benefit Gaza's residents.[50] Furthermore, the PA has been threatening to derail the ceasefire between Israel and Hamas, which could relieve some of the humanitarian pressures in Gaza and advance water and energy projects. The PA threatens to impose punitive measures on Gaza if the ceasefire does not meet the PA's conditions, delaying the prospects of some rehabilitation of Gaza.[51]

Given the dire situation in Gaza, it is clear that preventing a waterborne health disaster cannot wait until the different stakeholders find ways to overcome their differences. At the same time, it is important to acknowledge that successful adoption of many of our recommendations calls for creative thinking on how to operate within the complex political environment and address the various and daunting implementation challenges. We discuss four implementation issues and recommendations for addressing them: insufficient funding for WASH projects; limits on access and movement; the need for trusted networks and third-party mediation; and a required refocus on development of Gaza alongside emergency humanitarian aid. It is also criti-

[50] David Makovsky and Lia Weiner, "Hamas Failures in Gaza Are Changing Israel's Stance," *Times of Israel*, February 8, 2018.

[51] Entsar Abu Jahal, "Abbas Warns Hamas Against Potential Pact with Israel," *Al-Monitor*, September 5, 2018.

cal that stakeholders realize that, despite their importance in the long run, the completion of major infrastructure projects will take years, even under the most optimistic scenario; thus, while Israel, the PA, and donors advance these projects, stakeholders should prioritize short-term stabilization, mitigation measures, and steps aimed at preventing and responding to disease outbreaks (as detailed previously).

Enhance the Commitments of Donors who Pledged Funds for Major WASH Projects

The international community has been involved in Gaza for over two decades, providing funding for day-to-day services as well as major projects. In the WASH sector, projects require meaningful funding—e.g., the cost of the Gaza Central Desalination Plant is estimated at $560 million[52]—and donors have indeed pledged their support for such projects. Yet, in practice, history shows that donors regularly do not follow through on their commitments. One of the problems is that Gaza-centered donor conferences are structured as public events that pressure countries to increase their financial commitments for political gain, without a follow-through mechanism.[53]

Almost half of the $3.5 billion pledged in the Cairo conference, which followed the 2014 war between Israel and Hamas, had not been disbursed as of late March 2018.[54] Specifically, $13 million in funds for reconstruction of a destroyed hospital, $20 million for energy infrastructure, and $11 million for water infrastructure have not been provided as of March 2018.[55] Moreover, the 2017 $547 million Humanitarian Response Plan for the Palestinian Territories, most of it geared

52 European Commission, "Hope for Gaza: EU Creates Broad International Coalition to Provide Drinking Water to 2 Million People in Gaza," press release, Brussels, March 20, 2018.

53 Shira Efron and Ilan Goldenberg, "United States Policy Toward the Gaza Strip," in Anat Kurz, Udi Dekel, and Benedetta Berti, eds., *The Crisis of the Gaza Strip: A Way Out*, Tel Aviv: Institute for National Security Studies, 2017, pp. 165–181.

54 UNSCO, 2018a.

55 Office of the Quartet, 2018.

toward Gaza, was less than 50 percent funded, with the WASH cluster particularly underfunded.

Future projects are also hindered partially by funding gaps. For example, the Gaza Central Desalination Program still needed some $230 million to begin construction as of March 2018.[56] Even successful projects suffer from underfunding. For instance, a funding gap of $16.8 million was among the liabilities cited in mid-2018 jeopardizing NGEST's operations.[57]

Donors' reluctance to continue funding major projects in Gaza is grounded in four key concerns that cannot be addressed in the short term—the intra-Palestinian rivalry, continued limitations of access and movement imposed by Israel and Egypt, fear that investments in infrastructure would be eliminated in the next round of fighting between Hamas and Israel, and lack of proper governance in the energy and water sectors.[58] Donors are also reluctant to pay for maintenance and operations and for parts of projects that require investment inside Israel (e.g., the 161kV Line). First, despite challenges, it is important that donors fulfill their pledges for planning purposes and to avert a humanitarian crisis in Gaza. In addition, the donor community, Israel, and the PA should find creative ways to address existing funding gaps that are not yet bridged by pledges. As Israel actively seeks international funding for projects in Gaza,[59] experts have suggested that Israel should also consider joining the donor community, as it is in Israel's own interest to avert a humanitarian crisis in Gaza. Moreover, such a step could persuade other potential donors to increase their funding.[60]

It is crucial that additional funds and efforts be channeled to public health prevention measures, such as those outlined in our public

---

[56] Office of the Quartet, 2018.

[57] Office of the Quartet, 2018.

[58] World Bank, 2016.

[59] Josef Federman, "As Gaza Strip Deteriorates, Israel Turns to World for Help," *Times of Israel*, February 15, 2018.

[60] Conversation with a senior staff member of an NGO operating in Gaza, Los Angeles, February 5, 2018.

health recommendations, especially as such measures are less affected by political factors and can be advanced relatively quickly.

Relax Restrictions on Access and Movement

To implement many of these suggestions, the government of Israel will need to relax its strict restrictions on access and movement of goods through Kerem Shalom crossing, the only official crossing open for the transfer of goods into and out of Gaza,[61] which was shut down temporarily in July 2018 in response to attacks from Gaza using fire kites and incendiary balloons.[62] During 2017, Israel facilitated the approval of cement and rebar. Israel should similarly approve, simplify, and expedite the importation of additional items that are considered "dual-use." Israel could streamline its approval process to prevent delays in import approvals that hinder reconstruction, improvement of WASH facilities, and rehabilitation of the public health sector. The "dual-use" list is vague but, according to reports, as of September 2017, 4,000 items were pending approval before they could be imported,[63] and the list included 70 percent of the technical equipment needed for the WASH sector, such as pumps and chemicals for water purification.[64]

In February 2018, Israel and the PA agreed to jointly review the restrictions on the importation of dual-use items.[65] Furthermore, Israel approved in principle the entry of materials needed for water, wastewater, and WASH projects that the international community is seeking to advance. However, as of August 2018, the dual-use approval system has remained cumbersome and opaque. Even when approved, the entry of materials into Gaza needs to be coordinated and facilitated quickly and efficiently to allow for project implementation.[66] A strong level of inter-

[61] While, theoretically, imports could be made through Egypt, Cairo has kept Rafah, its border crossing with Gaza, mostly closed since 2014—and it is designed as a point of entry and exit for people rather than cargo.

[62] "Israel Cuts Gas, Fuel to Gaza as Egypt Shuts Rafah Gate," 2018.

[63] UNSCO, 2017.

[64] "Egypt Opens Border with Gaza Temporarily," 2018.

[65] UNSCO, 2018a.

[66] Conversation with UN official, Jerusalem, July 13, 2018.

national political engagement should be maintained to guarantee that Israel's commitment to support WASH projects will be translated into efficient and rapid processing of demands and that it will authorize the entry of required dual-use materials for these projects.

Israel has legitimate security concerns, but it should assess these security risks against the risk of a public health crisis in Gaza that would spill into Israel and for which the international community could hold Israel accountable. In parallel, the international community should address Egypt's security concerns stemming from terrorist networks in the Sinai Peninsula and ensure that Egypt more regularly opens Rafah, its only crossing with Gaza, which has been mostly closed since 2014.[67]

Identify Trusted Third Parties and Form International Coalitions

The lack of trust and competing agendas between the different parties (Hamas, the PA, Israel, Egypt, and the international community) and the constraints posed by Hamas's designation as a terrorist organization with which major donors do not interact has led to a need for creative mediation solutions. One such idea is forming a regional task force to implement immediate and mid-term responses to prevent or contain a disease outbreak. This would follow the example of groups like MECIDS but include representation from Gaza's medical sector.

In regard to energy, one of the barriers to the development of a viable energy sector is the Hamas-Fatah divide, and specifically their dispute over payments for electricity and transfer of collected fees. To address this problem, we propose two solutions. The first is that a trusted third party could act as an intermediary, coordinating between the factions and helping to advance meaningful solutions. The second idea is identifying potential solutions that could bypass the PA without engaging with Hamas in Gaza by funding, developing, and managing projects directly through private and international actors. We recognize that such a solution constitutes a serious political challenge for most Western donors and regional parties (including Egypt), who seek to empower the PA, Israel's partner in the peace process, and support

67 "Israel Cuts Gas, Fuel to Gaza as Egypt Shuts Rafah Gate," 2018.

its return to governance of Gaza while weakening Hamas. Still, if the intra-Palestinian dispute continues to hinder progress on major water and energy projects, there will be a need for creative thinking that could allow organizations like the UN to take the lead in all stages of project planning and implementation without sidelining the PA.[68]

Address Development Needs Alongside Humanitarian Relief

Given the emergency condition that persists in Gaza, it is only natural that attention is focused on humanitarian relief. Indeed, some of the criticism concerning proposed water and energy projects is that they will take years to complete and cannot stabilize Gaza and prevent a humanitarian crisis. At the same time, however, it is pivotal that alongside emergency response, which helps perpetuate aid dependency, the international community direct some of its efforts toward sustainable development that could alleviate Gaza's dependence on international assistance and help it become more self-sufficient.

Conclusion

Gaza is on the brink of a humanitarian collapse. One of the most alarming aspects of this crisis is an acute energy, water, and sanitation problem, which poses severe threats to public health.

In this report, we have detailed the linkages between the energy, water, sanitation, and public health issues in Gaza. In describing Gaza's water challenges, we specifically focused on water availability, quality, and affordability, as well as extremely limited access to wastewater treatment. In terms of threats to public health, we analyzed health issues that arise due to inadequate water quality (e.g., waterborne transmission of gastrointestinal disease, through both biological and chemical contamination) and inadequate water quantity and associated poor hygiene (e.g., contaminated food, hands, utensils, etc.). The risk of waterborne disease is exacerbated by poor infrastructure, limited

---

[68] Discussion with a former UN official who served in Gaza, Washington, D.C., June 4, 2018.

access to sufficient improved or clean water sources, and population density—conditions that characterize Gaza. Further, Gaza's young population is especially vulnerable to WASH-associated disease.

To address these challenges and prevent a health catastrophe, which could affect not only Gaza but also neighboring Egypt and Israel, we propose a set of recommendations that pertain to the energy, water, and public health sectors. The crisis in Gaza is manmade—a humanitarian rather than natural disaster—and solutions to many of the problems we describe are technical in nature. However, the barriers to adopting these recommendations are largely political, and hence we included a brief description of the political challenges and suggestions for overcoming them. At the same time, given the impact of political challenges and the difficulty in addressing them in the uniquely complex Gaza context, we indicate steps that all stakeholders could enact to help stabilize Gaza and prevent a humanitarian crisis that could spread well beyond its borders.

References

Abbas, Medhat, Maurizio Barbieri, Maria Battistel, Giuditta Brattini, Angelica Garone, and Barbara Parisse, "Water Quality in the Gaza Strip: The Present Scenario," *Journal of Water Resource and Protection*, Vol. 5, No. 1, 2013, pp. 54–63. As of August 16, 2018: http://file.scirp.org/pdf/JWARP_2013012511054871.pdf

Abu Amer, Ahmad, "Unpaid Gaza Employees Lash out at Qatari Ambassador," *Al-Monitor*, February 26, 2018.

Abu Amr, S. S., and Maged Mohammed Yassin, "Microbial Contamination of the Drinking Water Distribution System and Its Impact on Human Health in Khan Yunis Governorate, Gaza Strip: Seven Years of Monitoring (2000–2006)," *Public Health*, Vol. 122, No. 11, 2008, pp. 1275–1283.

Abu-Elamreen, F. H., A. A. Abed, and F. A. Sharif, "Viral, Bacterial and Parasitic Etiology of Pediatric Diarrhea in Gaza, Palestine," *Medical Principles and Practice*, Vol. 17, No. 4, 2008, pp. 296–301. As of August 16, 2018: https://www.karger.com/Article/Abstract/129609

Abu Jahal, Entsar, "Abbas Warns Hamas Against Potential Pact with Israel," *Al-Monitor*, September 5, 2018. As of September 28, 2018: http://www.al-monitor.com/pulse/originals/2018/08/palestinian-authority-abbas-threats-hamas-truce-israel.html#ixzz5RQBBlSHW

Aish, Adnan M., "Drinking Water Quality Assessment of the Middle Governorate in the Gaza Strip, Palestine," *Water Resources and Industry*, Vol. 4, 2013, pp. 13–20. As of August 16, 2018: https://www.sciencedirect.com/science/article/pii/S2212371713000413

Akram, Fares, "Desalination Plant Opens to Bring Gaza Some Relief," *Times of Israel*, January 19, 2017. As of March 10, 2018: https://www.timesofisrael.com/desalination-plant-opens-to-bring-gaza-some-relief/

Al Laham, Nahed, Mansour Elyazji, Rohaifa Al-Haddad, and Fouad Ridwan, "Prevalence of Enteric Pathogen-Associated Community Gastroenteritis Among Kindergarten Children in Gaza," *Journal of Biomedical Research*, Vol. 29, No. 1, 2015, pp. 61–68. As of August 16, 2018:
https://www.ncbi.nlm.nih.gov/pmc/articles/PMC4342437/

al-Mughrabi, Nidal, "Palestinian Authority Says Resuming Payment for Gaza's Israeli Electricity," Reuters, January 3, 2018a.

———, "UN Employees in Gaza Demonstrate Against U.S. Aid Cut," Reuters, January 28, 2018b. As of September 18, 2018:
https://www.reuters.com/article/us-israel-palestinians-usa-un/u-n-employees-in-gaza-hold-protest-strike-over-u-s-aid-cut-idUSKBN1FI1G7

———, "UAE, Qatar Donate Funds to Stave off Gaza Health Crisis," Reuters, February 9, 2018c.

Balousha, Hazem, "Israel Turns the Power Back on to Gaza, Giving Residents About Six Hours' Worth a Day," *Washington Post*, January 7, 2018

Ben Zikri, Almog, "Flammable Kites from Gaza Set Israeli Fields and Forests Ablaze," *Haaretz*, May 23, 2018. As of June 20, 2018:
https://www.haaretz.com/israel-news/.premium-flammable-kites-from-gaza-set-israeli-fields-and-forests-ablaze-1.6114230

Bromberg, Gidon, Giulia Giordano, Oded Eran, and Omri Elad, *The Water and Energy Crisis in Gaza: Snapshot 2017*, Tel Aviv: Institute for National Security Studies, 2017. As of March 10, 2018:
http://www.inss.org.il/publication/water-energy-crisis-gaza-snapshot-2017/

Cairncross, S., "More Water: Better Health," *People and the Planet*, Vol. 6, No. 3, 1997, pp. 10–11.

CMWU—*See* Coastal Municipalities Water Utility.

Coastal Municipalities Water Utility, *Damages Assessment Report, Water and Wastewater Infrastructure (Gaza Strip; July 7–August 14, 2014)*, August 2014. As of August 13, 2018:
https://www.humanitarianresponse.info/sites/www.humanitarianresponse.info/files/assessments/Damage_Assessment_Report_War%202014%20%28%20REV%201%29.pdf

"Communicable Diseases in the Gaza Strip—2016," General Directorate of Primary Health Care, Ministry of Health, Palestine, 2016.

Cravioto, Alejando, Claudio F. Lanata, Daniele S. Lantagne, and Balakrish Nair, *Final Report of the Independent Panel of Experts on the Cholera Outbreak in Haiti*, United Nations, 2011. As of August 15, 2018:
http://www.un.org/News/dh/infocus/haiti/UN-cholera-report-final.pdf

DeYoung, Karen, Ruth Eglash, and Hazem Balousha, "U.S. Ends Aid to United Nations Agency Supporting Palestinian Refugees," *Washington Post*, August 31, 2018. As of September 18, 2018:
https://www.washingtonpost.com/world/middle_east/us-aid-cuts-wont-end-the-right-of-return-palestinians-say/2018/08/31/8e3f25b4-ad0c-11e8-8a0c-70b618c98d3c_story.html?noredirect=on&utm_term=.3541fa8e35a7

Dheir, Majdi, and Nedal Ghuneim, *Communicable Diseases in Gaza Strip: Annual Report 2016*, Palestinian General Directorate of Primary Health Care Preventive Medicine, Epidemiology Department, September 2017. As of August 17, 2018:
http://www.moh.gov.ps/portal/wp-content/uploads/Annual-Epidemiological-Report-2016.pdf

EcoPeace Middle East, "Brief—Gaza's Water and Sanitation Crisis and Implications for Regional Stability," February 2016.

Efron, Shira, and Ilan Goldenberg, "United States Policy Toward the Gaza Strip," in Anat Kurz, Udi Dekel, and Benedetta Berti, eds., *The Crisis of the Gaza Strip: A Way Out*, Tel Aviv: Institute for National Security Studies, 2017, pp. 165–181.

"Egypt Opens Border with Gaza Temporarily," *The National*, February 21, 2018.

"Egypt Opens Gaza's Rafah Crossing for Ramadan," Associated Press, May 18, 2018. As of June 20, 2018:
https://www.voanews.com/a/egypt-opens-gaza-rafah-crossing-ramadan/4399514.html

Eisenbud, Daniel K., "World Bank to Help Fund Solar Panels Project in Gaza," *Jerusalem Post*, August 1, 2017. As of March 18, 2018:
http://www.jpost.com/Arab-Israeli-Conflict/World-Bank-to-help-fund-solar-panels-project-in-Gaza-501355

Eldar, Shlomi, "Gaza's Ticking Sewage Bomb," *Al-Monitor*, June 16, 2017. As of August 14, 2018:
https://web.archive.org/web/20170908042601/http://www.al-monitor.com/pulse/en/originals/2017/06/israel-gaza-strip-palestinians-elecrticity-ecology-water.html

Emergency Water, Sanitation, and Hygiene Group, "Life Under Blockade: 86% of Projects Necessary to Develop the Ravaged WASH Sector in Gaza Remain at Risk," press release, March 22, 2016. As of August 14, 2018:
https://web.archive.org/web/20170206134433/http://www.ewash.org/sites/default/files/inoptfiles/Press%20Release_EWASH%20World%20Water%20Day%20Palestine%202016_FNL.pdf

———, "Water and Sanitation in Palestine," fact sheet, 2017. As of August 14, 2018:
https://web.archive.org/web/20170911190106/http://www.ewash.org/sites/default/files/inoptfiles/160314%20-%20WATER%20AND%20SANITATION%20IN%20PALESTINE.pdf

Eran, Oded, Gidon Bromberg, and Michal Milner, *The Water, Sanitation and Energy Crises in Gaza: Humanitarian, Environmental and Geopolitical Implications with Recommendations for Immediate Measures*, Tel Aviv: EcoPeace Middle East, 2014.

Esrey, S. A., J. B. Potash, L. Roberts, and C. Shiff, "Effects of Improved Water Supply and Sanitation on Ascariasis, Diarrhoea, Dracunculiasis, Hookworm Infection, Schistosomiasis, and Trachoma," *Bulletin of the World Health Organization*, Vol. 69, No. 5, 1991, pp. 609–621. As of August 17, 2018: https://www.ncbi.nlm.nih.gov/pmc/articles/PMC2393264/

European Commission, "Giving Gaza Hope: Gaza Central Desalination Plant Providing Water to 2 Million People," fact sheet, undated. As of March 10, 2018: https://ec.europa.eu/neighbourhood-enlargement/sites/near/files/gaza_plant_factsheet.pdf

———, "Hope for Gaza: EU Creates Broad International Coalition to Provide Drinking Water to 2 Million People in Gaza," press release, Brussels, March 20, 2018. As of August 17, 2018:
http://europa.eu/rapid/press-release_IP-18-2081_en.htm

Fanack Water of the Middle East and North Africa, "Increasing Water Availability in Gaza," June 5, 2015.

Federman, Josef, "As Gaza Strip Deteriorates, Israel Turns to World for Help," *Times of Israel*, February 15, 2018. As of March 18, 2018:
https://www.timesofisrael.com/as-gaza-strip-deteriorates-israel-turns-to-world-for-help/

Fishman, Alex, "Israel Approves Solar Field to Increase Power Supply to Gaza," Ynet News, June 27, 2018. As of June 27, 2018:
https://www.ynetnews.com/articles/0,7340,L-5297677,00.html

Fry, L. M., J. R. Cowden, D. W. Watkins, Jr., T. Clasen, and J. R. Mihelcic, "Quantifying Health Improvements from Water Quantity Enhancement: An Engineering Perspective Applied to Rainwater Harvesting in West Africa," *Environmental Science & Technology*, Vol. 44, No. 24, 2010, pp. 9535–9541. As of August 17, 2018:
https://pubs.acs.org/doi/pdf/10.1021/es100798j

"Gaza in 2020: A Liveable Place?" press release, United Nations Relief and Works Agency for Palestine Refugees in the Near East, August 28, 2012. As of August 19, 2018:
https://www.unrwa.org/newsroom/press-releases/gaza-2020-liveable-place

"Gaza's Only Power Plant Stops Work Due to Lack of Fuel," *Middle East Monitor*, April 13, 2018. As of August 17, 2018:
https://www.middleeastmonitor.com/20180413-gazas-only-power-plant-stops-work-due-to-lack-of-fuel/

Ghuneim, Nedal, Majdi Dheir, and Khaled Abu Ali, "Epidemiology of Different Types of Meningitis Cases in Gaza Governorates, Occupied Palestinian Territory, December 2013–January 2014," *Journal of Antivirals & Antiretrovirals*, Vol. 8, No. 1, 2016, pp. 26–34. As of August 17, 2018:
https://www.omicsonline.org/open-access/epidemiology-of-different-types-of-meningitis-cases-in-gaza-governoratesoccupied-palestinian-territory-december-2013-january-2014-jaa-1000132.php?aid=70167

Gisha—Legal Center for Freedom of Movement, "Egyptian Power Supply Lines to Gaza to Resume Operations After Being Shut Down for Two Months," September 7, 2017. As of April 5, 2018:
http://gisha.org/updates/8198

Greenberg, Jonathan, "Trump's Decision to Cut UNRWA Funding Is the First Step Toward Middle East Peace," *Daily Wire*, January 17, 2018

Greenwald, Diana B., "Who Is Responsible for Solving Gaza's Massive Electricity Crisis?" *Washington Post*, February 5, 2018. As of April 4, 2018:
https://www.washingtonpost.com/news/monkey-cage/wp/2018/02/05/who-is-responsible-for-solving-gazas-massive-electricity-crisis/?noredirect=on&utm_term=.148f322308b2

Grossman, Michelle Malka, "Gaza Sewage Crisis Is a Ticking Timebomb for Israel," *Jerusalem Post*, March 17, 2016. As of August 17, 2018:
http://www.jpost.com/Arab-Israeli-Conflict/Gaza-sewage-crisis-is-a-ticking-timebomb-for-Israel-448335

Guidelines for Drinking Water Quality, Third Edition Incorporating the First and Second Addenda, Vol. 1: *Recommendations*, Geneva: World Health Organization, 2008. As of August 14, 2018:
http://www.who.int/water_sanitation_health/dwq/fulltext.pdf

Guidelines for Drinking Water Quality, Annex 5: Treatment Methods and Performance, 4th ed., Geneva: World Health Organization, 2011. As of August 16, 2018:
http://apps.who.int/iris/bitstream/handle/10665/44584/9789241548151_eng.pdf;jsessionid=0F3943F30467A6444B11477174BA47D9?sequence=1

Guttman, Nikki, "IDF Photos Prove Hamas Is Behind Gaza Kite Terrorism," *Israel Hayom*, June 26, 2018. As of June 26, 2018:
http://www.sun-sentinel.com/florida-jewish-journal/fl-jjps-kite-0704-20180626-story.html

Harris, Gardiner, "Trump Administration Cuts More Than $200 Million in Aid for Palestinians," *New York Times*, August 24, 2018. As of September 18, 2018:
https://www.nytimes.com/2018/08/24/us/politics/trump-palestinians-aid-cut.html

Husseini, Abdullatif, Niveen M. E. Abu-Rmeileh, Nahed Mikki, Tarik M. Ramahi, Heidar Abu Ghosh, Nadim Barghuthi, Mohammad Khalili, Espen Bjertness, Gerd Holmboe-Ottesen, and Jak Jervell, "Cardiovascular Diseases, Diabetes Mellitus, and Cancer in the Occupied Palestinian Territory," *The Lancet*, Vol. 373, No. 9668, 2009, pp. 1041–1049.

Inventory of Shared Water Resources in Western Asia, Beirut, Lebanon: United Nations Economic and Social Commission for Western Asia and German Federal Institute for Geosciences and Natural Resources, 2013.

"Israel Cuts Gas, Fuel to Gaza as Egypt Shuts Rafah Gate," *Daily Sabah*, July 17, 2018.

Khatib, Rasha, Rita Giacaman, Umaiyeh Khammash, and Salim Yusuf, "Challenges to Conducting Epidemiology Research in Chronic Conflict Areas: Examples from PURE-Palestine," *Conflict and Health*, Vol. 10, No. 1, 2016, p. 33.

Khoury, Jack, "Gaza on 4 Hours of Power a Day After Sole Electric Firm Shuts Down," *Haaretz*, February 22, 2018.

Liebermann, Oren, and Talal Abu Rahma, "Gaza Crippled by Electricity Crisis as Power Plant Runs out of Fuel," CNN, April 17, 2017. As of April 18, 2018: https://www.cnn.com/2017/04/17/middleeast/palestinians-gaza-power-plant-crisis/index.html

Liebermann, Oren, and Abeer Salman, "Israeli Mayors Call on US to Solve Gaza's Electricity Crisis," CNN, September 3, 2017.

Makovsky, David, and Lia Weiner, "Hamas Failures in Gaza Are Changing Israel's Stance," *Times of Israel*, February 8, 2018.

Manenti, Ambrogio, Claude de Ville de Goyet, Corinna Reinicke, John Macdonald, and Julian Donald, *Report of a Field Assessment of Health Conditions in the Occupied Palestinian Territory*, World Health Organization, February 2016. As of January 4, 2018:
http://apps.who.int/gb/Statements/Report_Palestinian_territory/Report_Palestinian_territory-en.pdf

McCasland, Margaret, Nancy M. Trautmann, Keith S. Porter, and Robert J. Wagenet, "Nitrate: Health Effects in Drinking Water," fact sheet, Ithaca, N.Y.: Cornell University Cooperative Extension. As of August 17, 2018:
http://psep.cce.cornell.edu/facts-slides-self/facts/nit-heef-grw85.aspx

Melhem, Ahmad, "Israeli-Palestinian Water Pact Raises Hopes, Suspicions," *Al-Monitor*, 2017. As of August 17, 2018:
https://www.marsad.ps/en/2017/07/25/israeli-palestinian-water-pact-raises-hopes-suspicions/

MICS—*See* "West Bank and Gaza—Multiple Indicator Cluster Survey 2014."

Middle East Consortium on Infectious Disease Surveillance, "Welcome Message," homepage, undated. As of March 23, 2018:
http://www.mecidsnetwork.org/

Milton-Edwards, Beverley, "Gaza Protests Highlight Humanitarian Crisis and Lack of Political Progress to Peace," Brookings, April 5, 2018. As of April 6, 2018:
https://www.brookings.edu/opinions/gaza-protests-highlight-humanitarian-crisis-and-lack-of-political-progress-to-peace/

Ministry of Education and Higher Education, United Nations Children's Fund in the State of Palestine, and Alpha International, "Water, Sanitation and Hygiene in Schools; Knowledge, Attitudes and Practices Survey: 2015–2016," December 2016. As of August 14, 2018:
https://www.unicef.org/oPt/UNICEF_-_English_Report_Final.pdf

Mitnick, Joshua, "Israel Approves Palestinian Move to Pressure Hamas with Electricity Cuts," *Los Angeles Times*, June 12, 2017. As of August 17, 2018:
http://www.latimes.com/world/middleeast/la-fg-israel-gaza-power-20170612-story.html

MoEHE—*See* Ministry of Education and Higher Education.

Moore, Melinda, "Cholera in Haiti: No Surprise This Time Around," *Inside Sources*, October 27, 2016.

Mordechai, Yoav (Poli), Michael Milstein, and Yotam Amitay, "The Next Gaza: The Gaza Strip Between a Dead End and a Glimmer of Hope," *Strategic Assessment*, Vol. 20, No. 3, October 2017. As of March 10, 2018:
http://www.inss.org.il/publication/next-gaza-gaza-strip-dead-end-glimmer-hope/

"Municipal Services in Gaza Reduced by 50%," *Middle East Monitor*, February 22, 2018.

Niezna, Maayan, *Hand on the Switch: Who's Responsible for Gaza's Infrastructure Crisis?* Tel Aviv–Jaffa, Israel: Gisha—Legal Center for Freedom of Movement, 2017. As of August 17, 2018:
http://gisha.org/UserFiles/File/publications/infrastructure/Hand_on_the_Switch-EN.pdf

"North Gaza Communities Will Finally Benefit from Sewage Treatment Services," World Bank, March 12, 2018. As of March 12, 2018:
http://www.worldbank.org/en/news/feature/2018/03/12/north-gaza-communities-will-finally-benefit-from-sewage-treatment-services

"Northern Gaza Emergency Sewage Treatment (NGEST) Project," fact sheet, World Bank, July 15, 2018. As of July 15, 2018:
http://projects.worldbank.org/P074595/northern-gaza-emergency-sewage-treatment-ngest-project?lang=en

OCHA—*See* United Nations Office for the Coordination of Humanitarian Affairs.

Office of the European Union Representative, "Water for Gaza: EU Switches on the Biggest Solar Energy Field in the Gaza Strip to Fuel Projects Providing Drinking Water to People in Dire Need," August 2, 2018. As of September 18, 2018:
https://eeas.europa.eu/delegations/palestine-occupied-palestinian-territory-west-bank-and-gaza-strip/49074/water-gaza-eu-switches-biggest-solar-energy-field-gaza-strip-fuel-projects-providing-drinking_en

Office of the Quartet, "Energy," fact sheet, undated. As of April 4, 2018:
http://www.quartetoffice.org/page.php?id=5e1e7ay6168186Y5e1e7a

———, *Report to the Ad Hoc Liaison Committee*, Brussels, March 20, 2018. As of April 4, 2018:
http://www.quartetoffice.org/files/OQ_AHLC_March_2018%20Report.pdf

Office of the United Nations Special Coordinator for the Middle East Peace Process, *Report to the Ad Hoc Liaison Committee*, New York, September 18, 2017.

———, "Nickolay Mladenov Special Coordinator for the Middle East Peace Process: Briefing to the Security Council on the Situation in the Middle East," January 25, 2018a.

———, *Report to the Ad Hoc Liaison Committee*, Brussels: United Nations, March 20, 2018b. As of August 26, 2018:
https://unsco.unmissions.org/sites/default/files/unsco_ahlc_report_-_march_2018_0.pdf

O'Reilly, Ciara E., Peter Jaron, Benjamin Ochieng, Amek Nyaguara, Jacqueline E. Tate, Michele B. Parsons, Cheryl A. Bopp, Kara A. Williams, Jan Vinjé, Elizabeth Blanton, Kathleen A. Wannemuehler, John Vulule, Kayla F. Laserson, Robert F. Breiman, Daniel R. Feikin, Marc-Alain Widdowson, and Eric Mintz, "Risk Factors for Death Among Children Less Than 5 Years Old Hospitalized with Diarrhea in Rural Western Kenya, 2005–2007: A Cohort Study," *PLoS Medicine*, Vol. 9, No. 7, July 3, 2012, p. e1001256. As of August 17, 2018:
http://journals.plos.org/plosmedicine/article?id=10.1371/journal.pmed.1001256

Palestine Economic Policy Research Institute, *Palestinian Economic Bulletin*, Bulletin 138, Portland Trust, March 2018. As of April 4, 2018:
http://a4vpe.org/documents/economic-reports/portland-trust/tpt-bulletin-issue-138-March-2018.pdf

Palestinian Central Bureau of Statistics, *Palestinian Multiple Indicator Cluster Survey 2014, Final Report*, Ramallah, Palestine, 2015. As of August 26, 2018:
https://mics-surveys-prod.s3.amazonaws.com/MICS5/Middle%20East%20and%20North%20Africa/State%20of%20Palestine/2014/Final/State%20of%20Palestine%202014%20MICS_English.pdf

———, *Palestine in Figures 2016*, Ramallah, Palestine, 2017. As of August 17, 2018:
http://www.pcbs.gov.ps/Downloads/book2261.pdf

———, "Palestinians' Population Status in the Palestine, 2016 (Arabic only)," State of Palestine, 2016.

Palestinian Central Bureau of Statistics, United Nations Children's Fund, and United Nations Population Fund, *Final Report of the Palestinian Family Survey 2010*, Ramallah, Palestine, 2013.

Palestinian Water Authority, "Gaza Strip: No Clean Drinking Water, No Enough Energy, and Threatened Future," fact sheet, 2014. As of August 17, 2018: https://web.archive.org/web/20151230104509/http://www.irinnews.org/pdf/pwa_gaza_water_fact_sheet_3-2014.pdf

———, "Terms of Reference for the Associated Works for Gaza Desalination Project," 2014.

"Palestinian Water Authority Announces Plans for Desalination Plant in Gaza," Ma'an News Agency, January 31, 2018. As of March 10, 2018: https://www.maannews.com/Content.aspx?id=779802

Palestinian Water Authority, Gruppo di Volontariato Civile–Italia, and United Nations Children's Fund, "WASH Assessment at the Household Level in the Gaza Strip," July 31, 2017. As of March 10, 2018: https://reliefweb.int/sites/reliefweb.int/files/resources/Gaza_WASH_HH_report_July2017_final.pdf

Palestinian Water Authority official, email exchange with authors, April 12, 2018.

Pandey, Pramod K., Philip H. Kass, Michelle L. Soupir, Sagor Biswas, and Vijay P. Singh, "Contamination of Water Resources by Pathogenic Bacteria," *AMB Express*, Vol. 4, No. 1, 2014, p. 51. As of August 15, 2018: https://www.ncbi.nlm.nih.gov/pmc/articles/PMC4077002/

Pomeranz, Avishalom, Ze'ev Korzets, Daniel Vanunu, Haim Krystal, and Baruch Wolach, "Elevated Salt and Nitrate Levels in Drinking Water Cause an Increase of Blood Pressure in Schoolchildren," *Kidney and Blood Pressure Research*, Vol. 23, No. 6, 200, pp. 400–403. As of August 17, 2018: https://www.ncbi.nlm.nih.gov/pubmed/11070420

"Population Growth in Occupied Palestinian Territory to Drive Demand for Housing, Services—UN," press release, UN News Center, December 21, 2016. As of August 19, 2018: https://news.un.org/en/story/2016/12/548332-population-growth-occupied-palestinian-territory-drive-demand-housing-services

Price, Yisrael, "Gaza Sewage Threatens Israel's Water Supply," *Hamodia*, March 21, 2016. As of January 4, 2017: https://hamodia.com/2016/03/21/gaza-sewage-threatens-israels-water-supply/

Protecting Children from Unsafe Water in Gaza: Strategy, Action Plan and Project Resources, Summary Documents, Ramallah: UNICEF–Occupied Palestine Territory, 2011. As of August 19, 2018: https://www.unicef.org/oPt/FINAL_Summary_Protecting_Children_from_unsafe_Water_in_Gaza_4_March_2011.pdf

PWA—*See* Palestinian Water Authority.

Ravid, Barak, "Netanyahu Wants to Transfer Part of UNRWA Funding to Jordan," Axios, March 8, 2018; conversation with Israel Defense Forces official, Tel Aviv, July 12, 2018.

Reed, Brian, and Bob Reed, "How Much Water Is Needed in Emergencies," Water, Engineering, and Development Centre, Loughborough University, Leiceistershire, UK, for World Bank, 2011. As of August 17, 2018: http://www.who.int/water_sanitation_health/publications/2011/tn9_how_much_water_en.pdf

"Report: 97% of Gaza's Drinking Water at Sewer Quality," JNi.Media, January 21, 2018.

"Report: Israel-Hamas Ceasefire Deal Nears Completion," Tazpit Press Service, August 24, 2018. As of September 18, 2018: https://www.breakingisraelnews.com/112820/israel-hamas-ceasefire-deal/

Shomar, Basem, Karsten Osenbrück, and Alfred Yahya, "Elevated Nitrate Levels in the Groundwater of the Gaza Strip: Distribution and Sources," *Science of the Total Environment*, Vol. 398, 2008, pp. 164–174. As of August 19, 2018: http://dx.doi.org/10.1016/j.scitotenv.2008.02.054

"Solar Power Brightens Gaza's Business Prospects," Environment News Service, March 15, 2018. As of August 17, 2018: http://ens-newswire.com/2018/03/15/solar-power-brightens-gazas-business-prospects/

State Comptroller, "Zihumei Mayim Bein Medinat Yisrael Le'Shitchey Yehuda, Shomron Ve'Aza [Water Pollutions Between the State of Israel and the Territories of Judea and Samaria and Gaza]," Publication of the Annual Report 67B, 2017, pp. 1481–1583. As of January 4, 2018: http://www.mevaker.gov.il/(X(1)S(dtuoybrn5lioxhnnsjixgyub))/he/publication/Articles/Pages/67b.aspx?AspxAutoDetectCookieSupport=1

Stelmach, R. D., and T. Clasen, "Household Water Quantity and Health: A Systematic Review," *International Journal of Environmental Research and Public Health*, Vol. 12, No. 6, 2015, pp. 5954–5974. As of August 19 2018: http://www.mdpi.com/1660-4601/12/6/5954/html

Tibon, Amir, and Amos Harel, "Trump Administration Will Ask Gulf States to Invest up to $1 Billion in Gaza Economy," *Haaretz*, June 17, 2018. As of June 17, 2018:
https://www.haaretz.com/us-news/.premium-trump-admin-wants-gulf-states-to-invest-up-to-1-billion-for-gaza-1.6180191

Tzuri, Matan, "Gaza Perimeter Agriculture in Peril Due to Water Reservoir Contamination," Ynet News, March 7, 2018.

Udasin, Sharon, "Cross-Border Water Pollution Threatens Israeli Security, Watchdog Says," *Jerusalem Post*, May 16, 2017. As of August 19, 2018:
http://www.jpost.com/Business-and-Innovation/Environment/Cross-border-water-pollution-threatens-Israeli-security-watchdog-says-490928

UN—*See* United Nations.

UNICEF—*See* United Nations Children's Fund.

United Nations, "Global Issues: Water," fact sheet, undated. As of August 14, 2018:
http://www.un.org/en/sections/issues-depth/water/

———, "Humanitarian Impact of the Gaza Electricity Crisis," fact sheet, May 2017a. As of January 30, 2018:
https://reliefweb.int/sites/reliefweb.int/files/resources/Gaza%20Electricity%20Crisis.pdf

———, *Gaza Ten Years Later*, July 2017b. As of August 14, 2018:
https://unsco.unmissions.org/sites/default/files/gaza_10_years_later_-_11_july_2017.pdf

United Nations Children's Fund, "Protecting Children from Unsafe Water in Gaza," June 10, 2010. As of August 19, 2018:
https://www.unicef.org/oPt/FINAL_C4D_Report_July_2010.pdf

———, "Immunization Country Profiles," database, July 2017. As of August 19, 2018:
https://data.unicef.org/resources/immunization-country-profiles-2/

United Nations Office for the Coordination of Humanitarian Affairs, "Occupied Palestinian Territory: Gaza Emergency Power Deficit (as of 21 August 2014)," ReliefWeb, August 21, 2014. As of August 19, 2018:
https://reliefweb.int/map/occupied-palestinian-territory/occupied-palestinian-territory-gaza-emergency-power-deficit-21

———, "The Humanitarian Impact of the Internal Palestinian Divide on the Gaza Strip," fact sheet, June 23, 2017a. As of August 19, 2018:
https://www.ochaopt.org/content/humanitarian-impact-internal-palestinian-divide-gaza-strip-june-2017

———, "Occupied Palestinian Territory: The Monthly Humanitarian Bulletin | July 2017," August 5, 2017b. As of August 19, 2018:
https://www.ochaopt.org/content/monthly-humanitarian-bulletin-july-2017

———, "OPt Humanitarian Fund Releases US $1 Million in Funds to Avoid Collapse of Services in the Gaza Strip; Additional Funds Needed Urgently," September 17, 2018. As of September 18, 2018:
https://www.ochaopt.org/content/opt-humanitarian-fund-releases-us1-million-funds-avoid-collapse-services-gaza-strip

United Nations Relief and Works Agency, "Occupied Palestinian Territory Emergency Appeal 2018," January 30, 2018.

UNRWA—*See* United Nations Relief and Works Agency.

UNSCO—*See* Office of the United Nations Special Coordinator for the Middle East Peace Process.

U.S. Centers for Disease Control and Prevention, "Ceramic Filtration," fact sheet, March 21, 2012a. As of August 17, 2018:
https://www.cdc.gov/safewater/ceramic-filtration.html

———, "Slow Sand Filtration," fact sheet, March 21, 2012b. As of August 16, 2018:
https://www.cdc.gov/safewater/sand-filtration.html

———, "Solar Disinfection," fact sheet, Atlanta, Ga., October 10, 2012c. As of August 19, 2018:
https://www.cdc.gov/safewater/solardisinfection.html

Water Resources Directorate, "2015 Water Resources Status Summary Report/ Gaza Strip," Ramallah: Palestinian Water Authority, 2016.

"Water Situation Alarming in Gaza," World Bank, November 22, 2016. As of August 14, 2018:
http://www.worldbank.org/en/news/feature/2016/11/22/water-situation-alarming-in-gaza

Weil, Ana A., Louise C. Ivers, and Jason B. Harris. "Cholera: Lessons from Haiti and Beyond," *Current Infectious Disease Reports*, Vol. 14, No. 1, 2012, pp. 1–8.

"West Bank and Gaza—Multiple Indicator Cluster Survey 2014," World Bank, 2014.

WHO—*See* World Health Organization.

WHO/UNICEF Joint Monitoring Programme, "Improved and Unimproved Water Sources and Sanitation Facilities," undated.

World Health Organization, "Chloride in Drinking-Water: Background Document for Development," 2003, originally published in *Guidelines for Drinking-Water Quality*, 2nd ed., Vol. 2: *Health Criteria and Other Supporting Information,* Geneva: World Health Organization, 1996. As of August 19, 2018: http://www.who.int/water_sanitation_health/dwq/chloride.pdf

———, "Rotavirus Vaccines: WHO Position Paper—January 2013," *Weekly Epidemiological Record*, Vol. 88, No. 5, February 1, 2013, pp. 49–64. As of August 19, 2018:
http://www.who.int/wer/2013/wer8805.pdf?ua=1

———, *Gaza Strip: Joint Health Sector Assessment Report*, prepared by the Health Cluster in the Occupied Palestinian Territory, Gaza, September 2014. As of August 19, 2018:
http://www.emro.who.int/images/stories/palestine/documents/Joint_Health_Sector_Assessment_Report_Gaza_Sept_2014-final.pdf

———, *Nitrate and Nitrite in Drinking-Water*, Revision 1, Geneva, July 1, 2016. As of August 19, 2018:
http://www.who.int/water_sanitation_health/dwq/chemicals/nitratenitrite2ndadd.pdf

———, "Cholera," fact sheet, February 1, 2018. As of August 19, 2018:
http://www.who.int/mediacentre/factsheets/fs107/en/

World Health Organization Working Group on Sodium, Chlorides, and Conductivity in Drinking-Water, *Sodium, Chlorides, and Conductivity in Drinking-Water: Report on a WHO Working Group, The Hague, 1–5 May 1978*, Copenhagen: World Health Organization Regional Office for Europe, 1979. As of August 14, 2018:
https://www.ircwash.org/sites/default/files/WHO-1978-Soduim.pdf

Zaanoun, Adel, "Death of Gazan Boy Puts Spotlight on Polluted Water," *Times of Israel*, August 26, 2017. As of August 19, 2018:
https://www.timesofisrael.com/death-of-gazan-boy-puts-spotlight-on-polluted-water/

Zaqoot, Hossam A., Mazen Hamada, and Mohammed A. El-Tabash, "Investigation of Drinking Water Quality in the Kindergartens of Gaza Strip Governorates," *Journal of Tethys*, Vol. 4, No. 2, 2016, pp. 88–99. As of August 19, 2018:
https://www.researchgate.net/publication/305577617_Investigation_of_drinking_water_quality_in_the_kindergartens_of_Gaza_Strip_Governorates

About the Authors

Shira Efron is a policy researcher at the RAND Corporation, a special advisor on Israel with RAND's Center for Middle East Public Policy, and a professor at the Pardee RAND Graduate School. She is leading RAND's new Israel program and researches issues related to Israel, the Middle East, food security, and technology adoption in the Middle East and Africa.

Jordan R. Fischbach is a senior policy researcher at the RAND Corporation, co-director of the Water and Climate Resilience Center, and an affiliate faculty member at the Pardee RAND Graduate School. He is a leader in climate adaptation, water resources management, and coastal planning.

Ilana Blum is a policy researcher whose work lies at the intersection of human security, international law, and gender dynamics of conflict. She has a master's in International Security Studies from the Fletcher School of Law and Diplomacy and previously worked at the RAND Corporation as a research assistant.

Rouslan I. Karimov is a doctoral candidate at the Pardee RAND Graduate School and an assistant policy researcher at RAND. Prior to RAND, he spent more than ten years as a statistics and monitoring specialist at UNICEF.

Melinda Moore is a senior physician policy researcher and associate director of the Population Health Program at the RAND Corporation. She is also a professor at the Pardee RAND Graduate School. She previously served with the Centers for Disease Control and Prevention for 20 years and the Department of Health and Human Services' Office Global Health Affairs (now Office of Global Affairs) for five years.